The advice I would give to young clinicians is the advice I was lucky enough to receive from a wonderful doctor and poet, William Carlos Williams. I accompanied him on his "house rounds" in the industrial cities of northern New Jersey, and he kept on saying this to me, and once he wrote it down: "Watch and listen and let these men and women and children, these patients, teach you, and they will (boy will they!)." Old Doc Williams he was called, and never did he fail to heed his own advice. He would say: "What's the matter?" Something in his face, his manner, his very soul, indicated that he meant the question. He got his answers—and did his best, thereafter, to earn the trust and confidence given him. "Technique is part of the game," he once told me, "but heart is what really matters." Yes, indeed.

Robert Coles, M.D.

Manual of Introductory Clinical Medicine

A Student-to-Student Guide

Second Edition

Roger M. Macklis, M.D.
Harvard Medical School, Class of 1983;
Instructor in Radiation Therapy, Harvard
Medical School; Staff Radiation Oncologist,
Joint Center for Radiation Therapy, Boston

Michael E. Mendelsohn, M.D.
Harvard Medical School, Class of 1982;
Fellow in Cardiology, Harvard Medical
School; Associate Physician, Brigham and
Women's Hospital, Boston

Gilbert H. Mudge, Jr., M.D.
Assistant Professor of Medicine,
Harvard Medical School; Director, Clinical
Cardiology Service, Brigham and Women's
Hospital, Boston
Faculty Editor

Foreword by Daniel D. Federman, M.D.
Professor of Medicine and
Dean for Students and Alumni,
Harvard Medical School

Little, Brown and Company
Boston / Toronto

To our parents and our patients

to our neighborhood patients.

Contents

Appendixes

Contributors from
the Clinical Faculty

Herbert L. Abrams, M.D.	Professor of Radiology, Stanford University School of Medicine, Stanford; Philip H. Cook Professor of Radiology, Emeritus, Harvard Medical School, Boston
Mark D. Altschule, M.D.	Honorary Curator of Prints and Photographic Collections, Francis Countway Library of Medicine; Consultant in Psychiatry, McLean Hospital, and Consultant in Medicine, Beth Israel Hospital, Boston
K. Frank Austen, M.D.	Theodore Bevier Bayles Professor of Medicine, Harvard Medical School; Chairman, Department of Rheumatology and Immunology, Brigham and Women's Hospital, Boston
Charles F. Barlow, M.D.	Bronson Crothers Professor of Neurology, Harvard Medical School; Neurologist-in-Chief, Department of Neurology, The Children's Hospital Medical Center, Boston
William Berenberg, M.D.	Professor of Pediatrics, Harvard Medical School; Director, Division of Cerebral Palsy, The Children's Hospital Medical Center, Boston
Eugene Braunwald, M.D.	Hersey Professor of the Theory and Practice of Physic, and Herrman Ludwig Blumgart Professor of Medicine, Harvard Medical School; Chairman and Physician-in-Chief, Department of Medicine, Brigham and Women's Hospital and Beth Israel Hospital, Boston
Turner E. Bynum, M.D.	Associate Professor of Medicine, Harvard Medical School; Director, Department of Clinical Gastroenterology, Brigham and Women's Hospital, Boston
J. Robert Cassady, M.D.	Associate Professor of Radiation Therapy, Harvard Medical School; Division Director, Department of Radiation Therapy, Joint Center for Radiation Therapy, The Children's Hospital Medical Center/Brigham and Women's Hospital, Boston

Cecil H. Coggins, M.D.	Associate Professor of Medicine, Harvard Medical School; Clinical Director, Renal Unit, Massachusetts General Hospital, Boston
Harvey J. Cohen, M.D.	Associate Professor of Pediatrics, Division of Pediatric Hematology/Oncology, The University of Rochester School of Medicine and Dentistry, Rochester, New York
Robert Coles, M.D.	Professor of Psychiatry and Medical Humanities, and Research Psychiatrist to Harvard University Health Services, Harvard University, Cambridge, Massachusetts
David M. Dawson, M.D.	Associate Professor of Neurology, Harvard Medical School; Senior Physician, Department of Neurology, Brigham and Women's Hospital, Boston
Roman W. DeSanctis, M.D.	Professor of Medicine, Harvard Medical School; Director, Clinical Cardiology, Massachusetts General Hospital, Boston
Lewis Dexter, M.D.	Professor of Medicine Emeritus, Harvard Medical School; Senior Physician, Cardiovascular Division, Brigham and Women's Hospital, Boston
Kenneth H. Falchuk, M.D.	Associate Professor of Medicine, Harvard Medical School; Physician, Brigham and Women's Hospital, Boston
Z. Myron Falchuk, M.D.	Associate Professor of Medicine, Harvard Medical School; Associate Physician, Department of Gastroenterology, Brigham and Women's Hospital, Boston
Thomas B. Fitzpatrick, M.D.	Edward Wigglesworth Professor and Chairman of Dermatology, Harvard Medical School; Chief, Dermatology Service, Massachusetts General Hospital, Boston
Norman Geschwind, M.D.*	James Jackson Putnam Professor of Neurology, Harvard Medical School; Director, Department of Neurology, Beth Israel Hospital, Boston
Warren E. Grupe, M.D.	Associate Professor of Pediatrics, Harvard Medical School; Director, Pediatric Nephrology, The Children's Hospital Medical Center, Boston

* Deceased

Leston L. Havens, M.D.	Professor of Psychiatry, Harvard Medical School; Senior Staff Psychiatrist, The Cambridge Hospital, Cambridge, Massachusetts
Harley A. Haynes, M.D.	Associate Professor of Dermatology, Harvard Medical School; Director, Department of Dermatology, Brigham and Women's Hospital, Boston
Samuel Hellman, M.D.	Physician-in-Chief, Memorial Hospital, New York City
Roland H. Ingram, Jr., M.D.	Parker B. Francis Professor of Medicine, Harvard Medical School; Director, Respiratory Division, Brigham and Women's Hospital and Beth Israel Hospital, Boston
Homayoun Kazemi, M.D.	Professor of Medicine, Harvard Medical School; Chief, Pulmonary Unit, Massachusetts General Hospital, Boston
Stephen M. Krane, M.D.	Professor of Medicine, Harvard Medical School; Chief, Arthritis Unit, Massachusetts General Hospital, Boston
Jeffrey M. Lipton, M.D.	Assistant Professor of Pediatrics, Harvard Medical School; Assistant Physician, Dana Farber Cancer Institute, and Associate Physician, Department of Hematology, Brigham and Women's Hospital, Boston
Henry J. Mankin, M.D.	Edith M. Ashley Professor of Orthopedic Surgery, Harvard Medical School; Chief, Department of Orthopedic Surgery, Massachusetts General Hospital, Boston
Robert P. Masland, Jr., M.D.	Associate Professor of Pediatrics, Harvard Medical School; Chief, Division of Adolescent/Young Adult Medicine, The Children's Hospital Medical Center, Boston
Donald N. Medearis, Jr., M.D.	Charles R. Wilder Professor of Pediatrics, Harvard Medical School; Chief, Children's Service, Massachusetts General Hospital, Boston
Francis D. Moore, M.D.	Moseley Professor of Surgery Emeritus, Harvard Medical School; Surgeon-in-Chief Emeritus, Peter Bent Brigham Hospital, Boston
Gilbert H. Mudge, Jr., M.D.	Assistant Professor of Medicine, Harvard Medical School; Director, Clinical Cardiology Service, Brigham and Women's Hospital, Boston

Alexander S. Nadas, M.D.	Professor of Pediatrics, Harvard Medical School; Chief Emeritus, Department of Cardiology, The Children's Hospital Medical Center, Boston
David G. Nathan, M.D.	Robert A. Stranahan Professor of Pediatrics, Harvard Medical School; Pediatrician-in-Chief, Dana Farber Cancer Institute, and Chief, Division of Hematology/Oncology, The Children's Hospital Medical Center, Boston
Henning Pontoppidan, M.D.	Professor of Anesthesia, Harvard Medical School; Medical Director, Department of Respiratory Care and Respiratory Intensive Care Unit, Massachusetts General Hospital, Boston
John T. Potts, Jr., M.D.	Jackson Professor of Clinical Medicine, Harvard Medical School; Chief, General Medicine Services, Massachusetts General Hospital, Boston
Arnold S. Relman, M.D.	Professor of Medicine, Harvard Medical School; Editor, *New England Journal of Medicine*
Stephen H. Robinson, M.D.	Professor of Medicine, Harvard Medical School; Chief, Hematology Unit, and Clinical Director, Department of Medicine, Beth Israel Hospital, Boston
Edwin W. Salzman, M.D.	Associate Professor of Surgery, Harvard Medical School; Visiting Surgeon, Beth Israel Hospital, Boston
Arthur A. Sasahara, M.D.	Professor of Medicine, Harvard Medical School; Chief, Medical Services, West Roxbury Veterans Administration Medical Center, Boston
J. Gordon Scannell, M.D.	Clinical Professor of Surgery, Harvard Medical School; Senior Surgeon, Massachusetts General Hospital, Boston
John Shillito, Jr., M.D.	Professor of Surgery, Harvard Medical School; Associate Chief, Department of Neurosurgery, The Children's Hospital Medical Center, Boston
William Silen, M.D.	Johnson and Johnson Professor of Surgery, Harvard Medical School; Surgeon-in-Chief, Department of Surgery, Beth Israel Hospital, Boston
Eve E. Slater, M.D.	Senior Director, Department of Biochemical Endocrinology, Merck Sharpe & Dohme Research Laboratories, West Point, Pennsylvania

Thomas W. Smith, M.D.	Professor of Medicine, Harvard Medical School–Massachusetts Institute of Technology Division of Health Sciences and Technology; Chief, Cardiovascular Division, Brigham and Women's Hospital, Boston
Thomas P. Stossel, M.D.	Professor of Medicine, Harvard Medical School; Chief, Hematology/Oncology Unit, Massachusetts General Hospital, Boston
Marshall A. Wolf, M.D.	Associate Professor of Medicine, Harvard Medical School; Associate Physician-in-Chief, Department of Medicine, Brigham and Women's Hospital, Boston

Foreword

Ever since Hippocrates, physicians have sworn to teach their art to younger persons anxious to become doctors. The word *doctor* means "teacher," and our traditional image of the role is based on the bearded, flowing-robed master himself. Through the years, the physician-teacher has remained a venerable figure, and down to modern times we find senior physicians, rich in clinical experience, teaching their art.

But times have changed. Good medicine now is a remarkable blend of science, technology, skill, and humanism. Much of the education of medical students takes place in a curious temple, the teaching hospital, where priest and acolyte can barely be distinguished. Junior faculty and resident physicians are important members of the teaching staff. Indeed, many features of medical education make younger people important members of the teaching team. The social contract between patient and physician is an extraordinary one, incorporating a ready intimacy and deep candor unknown in any other human interaction. The student physician has to honor this personal expectation while simultaneously learning new skills and recalling a wealth of basic science. Although senior physicians often seem to forget how difficult and threatening this early clinical experience can be, sensitive house staff and senior students can convey the lessons to their juniors with particular effectiveness. In addition, many students are so apprehensive about evaluations that they hide their insecurities and uncertainties from senior physicians, who are allowed to peek through only with younger colleagues.

It is these changes and challenges in learning medicine that set the stage for this book, the work of two tyros barely bearded and certainly not venerated—at least until now. Is it surprising that two medical students should be offering advice about how to be a good medical student? Hardly, for students have always turned to those just ahead of them and this book is in essence a systematic set of answers to the questions of novices. Is it impious for novitiates to put their mark on the tablets? Not at all, for medicine now incorporates the novelty and irreverence of science with the traditions of clinical care. But can *all* the teaching be left to the young? By no means: Macklis and Mendelsohn had the help of an outstanding clinical teacher, Dr. Gilbert Mudge, as well as a bounteous harvest of insights and guidance from a large and diverse group of senior faculty.

In this book, then, two bright and dedicated student-physicians have reached out both to honor Hippocrates and to help their peers. The result is a first-rate guide for medical students entering their clinical years.

Daniel D. Federman

Preface to the Second Edition

It has been five years since the *Manual of Introductory Clinical Medicine* was first written. In that time, there have been some dramatic changes in medicine: The widespread use of magnetic resonance imaging has allowed new anatomic definition of a wide variety of disorders; the proliferation of new cardiovascular and antibiotic medications has increased the degree of pharmacologic intervention in patients with cardiac and infectious diseases; organ transplantation has become more routine; and a new, virally transmitted disease has threatened to become the plague of our century.

Despite these changes, the process by which a medical student moves from the classroom to the wards remains essentially unchanged. The physical examination and essential laboratory testing that constitute the basic medical work-up are identical. The intentional lack of a therapeutic emphasis in this manual, along with the essentially unchanged approach to the medical work-up, leaves many sections relatively unchanged. New material on AIDS, the breast examination, and the off-service note has been added, as have color illustrations of the dermatologic lesions and Gram stain findings that are frequently encountered during the clinical experience. Most sections have been rewritten in part, but we have deliberately avoided temptations to rewrite the book from an attending physician's point of view. We believe that the manual still presents a student-to-student perspective and hope that medical students continue to find it useful.

R. M. M.
M. E. M.
G. H. M.

Preface to the First Edition

This is a book written by medical students for medical students. It is addressed to students undergoing the most difficult part of their medical school training—the six or eight months that serve as the transition between the preclinical years and advanced clinical work. For most students, this period begins with instruction in the essentials of patient interviewing and physical diagnosis and proceeds through the first few months of the core clinical rotations. Although for many students this stage of medical school is the most exciting, it is also the most difficult. It is the period that the majority of us will remember most vividly when we think about medical school.

Why is the transition so difficult? It is not simply the amount of new material to be learned, for we have all spent late nights memorizing tedious material during our preclinical years. Nor is it simply the number of hours spent at the desk and bedside; long hours are nothing new for us. Rather, it is the shift in emphasis from the theoretical and academic to the practical and mundane that makes the transition period such an anxious time. Students have spent close to two years learning textbook medicine; suddenly they are confronted with the world of real illness, with patients and house officers and nurses and lab tests and requisition forms and bloods that must be drawn. During the preclinical years, they were expected to be university scholars. Now they are expected to be trade-school apprentices learning the nuts and bolts of their future craft.

An air of excitement and some measure of anxiety mark the transition from the preclinical to clinical years. The anxiety may be openly expressed or hidden by a white coat of cultivated sophistication. It may range from passive bewilderment to uncomfortable levels of assertiveness. You are leaving the tidy world of the library, the seminar, and the laboratory to face the infinite variations of illness and the human condition. You are a student and something more; you are a doctor and something less. You are no longer merely a spectator; as an observer you become part of another person's life, for good or ill. You will find that Hippocrates had something in that old aphorism, "The art is long, decision difficult." You will make mistakes that others will forgive but you will remember.

You have weathered many years of academic competition; now for these last all too brief years of medical school, enjoy what you have earned. If you feel too put upon, take some time for yourself. Remember Kipling's words about a doctor's work: "It seems to be required of you that you must save others. It is nowhere laid down that you need save yourselves."

J. Gordon Scannell, M.D.

Medicine is a transaction between two persons—a patient and a doctor—and hence is more process than content. The process is affected by local factors, but regardless of time and place it has basically uniform characteristics. It is both valid and useful to study the medical practices of other times and places. The content of medicine is highly variable and much of it is superstitious—the amount of superstition depending not only on the degree of ignorance, but also on the amount of data. The content can change markedly and rapidly, but the basic processes change slowly.

Mark D. Altschule, M.D.

This manual was compiled by two second-year medical students who had recently undergone this transition. It was written with two major goals in mind. First, it attempts to present a brief, telegraphic compilation of some of the factual material that the novice clinician should have at hand as he or she begins work in the hospital. This material includes both specific information on the content and performance of patient work-ups and more general information on the pathophysiology and differential diagnosis of about fifty common diseases with which the student will be confronted in the course of general medical rotations. This practical information, culled from our texts and notes, represents a selection and organization of the core material that we wish had been given to us at the beginning of our ward work. All of this information is available elsewhere in much longer, more detailed form, and this book is in no sense a substitute for these more authoritative texts. Yet in our experience the novice clinician is often overwhelmed by reference books that try to teach everything at once, books that in their attempt to be comprehensive do not succeed in instilling a sense of what is truly core material and what is less essential. Our hope in compiling this manual is that once a student has mastered the basics presented here, the more comprehensive treatments will be more accessible and more useful.

Second, because we believe that the student's transition-period anxiety stems in large part from an insecurity about the practical aspects of clinical work, we have appended to each chapter dealing with the medical work-up a brief discussion of the pragmatic issues that confront a student on the wards. These collections of clinical tips and practical points cover the same basic material as the factual information but approach it from a different angle. The practical information is highly subjective and somewhat idiosyncratic, but it is presented here because it represents an informal set of student-to-student tips that we wish had been available to us at the start of our clerkships.

To supplement our student-to-student tips, we canvassed a group of about one hundred of the attending physicians at Harvard Medical School selected on the basis of their reputations as excellent clinical teachers. We asked them to write a few sentences of advice, either practical or philosophical, directed toward medical students just beginning their clinical work. The "clinical pearls" found throughout this book are their responses to our open-ended request. Space considerations prevented us from publishing them all.

Once again, we emphasize that this manual is not a textbook but rather an organized compilation of factual material, practical information, and clinical tips meant to give medical students a head start in their clinical work. A few evenings with this book will teach the student much of the material that he or she would ordinarily acquire only after months on the wards. It is meant to be a truly student-oriented introduction to clinical medicine.

R. M. M.
M. E. M.
G. H. M.

Acknowledgments

We continue to be indebted to our classmates, colleagues, and teachers at the Harvard Medical School. We also are grateful to the staff at Little, Brown and Company, and especially to Susan Pioli for her continual advice and expertise in the preparation of this second edition. Punky Mudge provided us with help and encouragement throughout the project. Finally, Anne and Carol and our families continue to provide the understanding and support necessary to allow us to participate in modern academic medicine.

R. M. M.
M. E. M.

Acknowledgments

We wish to thank our colleagues...

I The Medical Work-Up

The *medical work-up* is a term used to refer to the sequence of diagnostic inquiries and laboratory tests that are implemented during the evaluation of any specific medical problem. The primary job of the medical student starting clinical work is to become familiar with the work-up process and to learn to conduct a patient work-up thoroughly and efficiently.

Although the specific details of the work-ups for various problems may be quite different, the **sequence of data acquisition and analysis** is always the same: fiirst a **history** is taken, then a **physical examination** is performed, then the **laboratory data** are collected and analyzed, and finally the **diagnostic and therapeutic plan** is formulated. This sequence of history–physical examination–laboratory data–assessment–plan is the heart of every work-up.

Part I of this book is organized in a sequence roughly parallel to that of the work-up. The first chapter outlines the content and technique of the **medical interview,** while the second chapter presents an outline of the general **physical examination.** A collection of eponymic physical exam signs and some key surface anatomy drawings are included as appendices to this chapter. Because the cardiovascular examination is perhaps the most difficult of the organ system evaluations, a more detailed treatment of this portion of the physical exam is presented in Chap. 3.

Turning from the bedside work-up to the clinical laboratory, the next six chapters present brief overviews of the principles and interpretation of the six most common laboratory tests: the **hematologic screen,** the **serum chemistry battery,** the **chest x-ray,** the **electrocardiograph,** the **urinalysis,** and the **arterial blood gas determination.** In each of these chapters, an attempt has been made to simplify the interpretation of the lab results and to concentrate only on the more common and significant findings. These chapters do not, of course, take the place of the more rigorous treatments found elsewhere.

Chap. 10 is a discussion of the **medical case write-up,** and includes a sample student write-up as well as specific advice on how a good write-up is constructed. The **medical case presentation** is described in Chap. 11, which contains specific advice on how to present medical cases on hospital rounds and in formal didactic sessions.

Because the information in all of these chapters is of two types, objective and subjective, each chapter is divided into two parts. Part A contains generally objective information that will be useful as a memory aid and as an easily accessible pocket reference. Part B contains subjective advice and pragmatic information that traditionally has been passed informally from student to student; its purpose is to help students "learn the ropes" of clinical work early in their careers in order to give them more time to concentrate on the factual information that must be mastered. As much as possible, Parts A and B of each chapter parallel each other and should be read together.

This book contains no specific therapeutic information; for this the student is referred to the *Manual of Medical Therapeutics* (also published by Little, Brown and Company). For the novice clinician this latter book is indispensable.

The Bedside Work-Up

"Listen to the patient. He will tell you the diagnosis." This well-known admonition of Dr. Hermann Blumgart to generations of medical students underscores the importance of an empathetic and sensitive history, but the patient will teach the receptive physician more than the simple identity of his illness. Given a prepared and responsive listener, the patient will also reveal for his examiner the most intimate workings of his disease process. A sick patient is an experiment of nature. The sapient clinician must reserve one corner of his mind for clues the patient will provide to unresolved questions about his disorder. The patient who manifests an unusual feature of his illness, no matter how humdrum the diagnosis, or the patient who presents with an uncommon diagnosis, or the patient with a mystifying illness and no clear diagnosis—any of these may provide the acute observer with new understanding of a previously stubborn and frustrating question. The patient is prepared to teach professor and student alike; they must be prepared to be his pupils.

Edwin W. Salzman, M.D.

1   The Patient Interview

The patient interview, usually referred to as the *history,* is the first step in the diagnostic work-up. Taking a good history is probably the single most important task in the work-up both because of its importance in diagnosis and because the history is the portion of the work-up in which the physician-patient relationship is first established. The job of the medical student is not only to learn how to conduct a thorough interview but also to develop a professional manner that will put the patient at ease while doing so. Whether the patient regards the student as an unnecessary third party or as a vital member of the medical team often depends on the tenor and style of the initial interview.

Part A of this chapter is a point-by-point review of the subjects and style of each part of the formal medical interview. Part B contains a collection of practical advice intended to help the student conduct and interpret the interview.

The parts of the medical interview that should be memorized early in the clinical career are outlined in Table 1-1. Chap. 10 presents information and formats useful in subsequently writing up the case for the medical record.

The interview is often neglected and poorly taught as it pertains to internal medicine: *learn to distinguish the interview from the history* (and recognize where they overlap) and, while interviewing, listen to the patient. Allow the first part of the interview to be as associative in character as possible; use interrogation later or only sparingly to aid a reticent patient or to restrict the rare patient who is rambling and circumstantial.

Turner E. Bynum, M.D.

It is virtually impossible to communicate with patients too much. Patients who understand the nature of their ailments and the objectives of their therapy deal with their illnesses more intelligently, and can make the physician's job easier. In the hospital, most communication occurs at the time of the *the daily visit.* No matter how busy he or she becomes, the physician should never forget that the highlight of any patient's day consists of the few moments when the doctor drops by. The daily visit should be as sacrosanct to the physician as it is to the patient.

Roman W. DeSanctis, M.D.

Table 1-1. The patient interview: The history and review of systems

 I. Introductory information
 II. Chief complaint and its duration
 III. History of the present illness
    A. Symptom analysis
    B. Review of pertinent systems
    C. Concluding the history of the present illness
 IV. Past medical history
    A. Other medical problems
    B. Allergies
    C. Major childhood illnesses
    D. Immunizations
    E. Injuries, hospitalizations, and operations
 V. Family history
    A. Family members
    B. Specific inheritable diseases
 VI. Psychosocial history
    A. Lifestyle
    B. Homelife
    C. Occupational life
       1. Nature of work
       2. Toxic exposures
    D. Sexual history
 VII. Medications and habits
    A. Medications
    B. Habits
 VIII. Review of systems
 IX. Conclusion of the history

A   **The History and Review of Systems**

 I. **Introductory information.** Begin by collecting the identifying data about a patient from both the existing medical record and the patient. This information includes especially the patient's name, age, sex, race, and occupation, as well as his place of birth, marital status, religion, and, if the patient has been referred from elsewhere, the source and reason for the referral. The introductory information is an important beginning from an administrative as well as diagnostic viewpoint.

 II. **Chief complaint and its duration.** The chief complaint is traditionally defined as that problem or set of problems that makes the patient decide to seek medical attention. Questions concerning the chief complaint follow the physician's greeting of the patient (see Part B, sec. **I.E**) and the brief questions about introductory information; they open that portion of the interview devoted to the present illness. The chief complaint is elicited by asking an open-ended question such as "What made you decide to come to the hospital?," "What brings you here today?," or "What seems to be the trouble?"

 The **duration** of the chief complaint provides an important temporal framework for the physician and should be inquired about and considered at this time.

 III. **History of the present illness.** The logical continuation and expansion of the chief complaint is the history of the present illness (HPI). The HPI is told by the patient to the interviewer who is predominantly a listener at this point of the interview, interjecting questions or phrases that may facilitate the flow of information when appropriate.

Table 1-2. Symptom analysis

Dimension	Typical question	Synonyms and related ideas
1. Location	Where is the pain located?	Main site, region, radiation
2. Quality	What is it like?	Character
3. Quantity	How intense is it?	Severity, frequency, periodicity, degree of functional impairment
4. Chronology	When did it begin and what course has it followed?	Onset, duration, frequency, periodicity, temporal characteristics
5. Setting	Under what circumstances does the pain take place?	Relation to physiologic functions
6. Aggravating-alleviating factors	What, if anything, makes the pain worse or better?	Provocative-palliative factors
7. Associated manifestations	What other symptoms or phenomena are associated with this pain?	Effects of disease, related concerns

A. **Symptoms.** The crux of the HPI is a detailed exploration of the symptoms that constitute the chief complaint. It is during this portion of the interview that the physician begins to engage in more active questioning. Each symptom should be investigated thoroughly by first listening to the patient's unfolding story and then questioning specifically to discover any dimensions of the symptoms that may have been omitted. One version of the specific dimensions of the symptom to be explored is detailed in Table 1-2.

B. **Review of pertinent systems.** The chief complaint and HPI usually suggest the involvement of one or more organ systems in the patient's illness. It is useful to inquire about each Review of Systems topic that relates to the organ systems involved while discussing the present illness. This implies that inferences about the disease process must be made during the history-taking procedure (probable organ systems involved must be identified). It is also therefore necessary to be familiar with the Review of Systems topics for the various organ systems in order to review the pertinent systems during the HPI (see Table 1-3). The purpose of reviewing the pertinent organ systems at this point is to accumulate further support for or evidence against diagnoses being considered by the interviewer. For example, if a patient enters with a chief complaint of "spitting blood," the interviewer will inquire about each topic in the Respiratory Systems review. It then becomes diagnostically useful to note a recent history of TB exposure (a pertinent positive); and it is also helpful to discover that the patient does not smoke (a pertinent negative).

C. **Concluding the HPI** with a question that gives the patient a further chance to air concerns (e.g., "Is there anything else about these recent pains that you would like to bring up?") completes this portion of the interview.

IV. **Past medical history.** The past medical history (PMH) portion of the interview logically follows the HPI. This portion of the interview is devoted to defining and describing medical problems that may be related to the present illness, problems that are active but unrelated to the HPI, and problems that existed at one time but are inactive at present. Although some patients may remember and provide much of the information during this part of the interview, portions of the past medical history are often discovered in and elaborated by the existing medical record. The past medical history includes questions about medical problems other than the present illness, allergies, childhood illnesses, immunizations, injuries, hospitalizations, and operations.

A. Other medical problems are sought by the interviewer, with a particular effort toward discovering any existing medical problems that may relate to the present illness. For instance, a 10-year history of hypertension may be of particular interest in a patient who enters complaining of chest pain. Note that these "other medical problems" may have been identified during the review of pertinent systems (see sec. **III. B**). However, it is at this point of the interview that a brief summary of the patient's problems is constructed. The interview for other problems should include questions concerning date of onset, diagnostic procedures, and major therapy for the problem in question. For each medical problem discovered it is also important to gain an understanding of the current status of the problem. For the patient with hypertension mentioned above, it would be important to inquire about how well the hypertension has been controlled since its diagnosis and treatment 10 years ago and to ask for the most recent blood pressure measurement. In inquiring about other medical problems a list that includes both active and inactive problems will often be generated.

B. Allergies should be documented carefully. The patient should be specifically questioned about drug reactions and reactions to prior blood transfusions or hospital procedures. When a patient notes an allergy, it is extremely important to obtain a description of the specific allergic reaction. Is a penicillin allergy manifested with a rash on the upper trunk or with spasm of the larynx and difficulty breathing?

C. Major childhood illnesses such as tuberculosis, rheumatic or scarlet fever, or polio should be investigated.

D. Injuries, hospitalizations, and operations are also sought in this portion of the interview. Included is any history of auto or other accidents, broken bones, trauma, or surgery. Previous hospital admissions should be sought, and the reason for the admission, the date and year, and the hospital involved should be systematically explored.

E. Immunizations for polio, measles, mumps, diphtheria, pertussis, tetanus, and so on are inquired about in the PMH portion of the patient interview, especially in pediatric patients.

V. Family history. The history turns to questions about the family after the patient's medical problems have been explored. This part of the interview has two goals: to find out about the health of immediate family members, and to discover whether certain common diseases with a familial pattern exist.

A. The age and health of the patient's parents, siblings, spouse, and children are first discussed. If a family member is deceased, the cause of death is noted.

B. The occurrence of any disease like that described in the patient's HPI is sought in other family members. Important diseases with a strong hereditary component or tendency for family clustering are also sought, including coronary artery disease, heart disease, diabetes mellitus, high blood pressure, stroke, asthma, allergies, arthritis, anemia, cancer, kidney disease, or mental illness.

VI. Psychosocial history. Although some of the information sought in this portion of the interview emerges from simply speaking with the patient while taking the history, several goals exist for the psychosocial history. Specifically, insights into the patient's lifestyle, homelife, occupational life, and attitude toward the disease and the hospitalization are sought. This is also the portion of the interview in which many physicians choose to take the sexual history (see **D**).

A. Lifestyle. An attempt should be made to understand what constitutes a typical day for the patient, what recreation the patient engages in and what religious beliefs he or she holds. The patient's school and military experience may be inquired into at this point.

B. Homelife. Housing, emotional atmosphere at home, marriage and family, and significant others should be briefly explored. An attempt should be made to identify factors that have influenced the relation between the patient's disease and homelife. Such questions may range from concerns about the physical layout of the home to the impact of the disease on the family.

C. Occupational life. Two goals exist for this portion of the psychosocial history. First, the nature of the patient's occupation is explored, and second, when relevant, the likelihood of a toxic exposure related to the patient's job is investigated.

1. **Nature of the occupation** is evaluated through asking what the patient does for work and attempting to gain insight into the relative satisfactions and dissatisfactions associated with work and the workplace.

2. **Toxic exposures** may be especially relevant in patients with respiratory or dermatologic disease without obvious etiology (e.g., silicosis in a cement plant worker or contact dermatitis on a surgeon's face or hands). Occupational exposures may occasionally be associated with disease of the liver (e.g., hepatitis in a hospital worker), central nervous system (e.g., polyneuropathy in an insecticide worker), or other organ systems. Exposures may also play a role in oncologic illness (mesothelioma in a shipyard worker with brief asbestos exposure or hematologic malignancy in a worker exposed to radiation).

D. Sexual history. Either at this point in the interview or during the genitourinary portion of the Review of Systems, the sexual history may be sought. It should include an attempt to evaluate the patient's attitude toward his or her sex life and a search for current or recently emerging difficulties. The sexual history is particularly important in cases with possible venereal, gynecologic, or psychologic problems (e.g., a woman with a chronic vaginal discharge may be far more upset by the effect that her difficulties have had on her sexual life than about the disease itself). The sexual history is also relevant to patients with chronic, debilitating disease that may interfere with the normal sex life of the patient. Some male patients, for example, find that the most disturbing aspect of a chronic disease such as diabetes mellitus is the impotence sometimes associated. Although this is a traditionally difficult portion of the interview (see Part B, **VI**), a simple inquiry as to whether or not the patient finds his or her sexual life satisfying often suffices to initiate the discussion.

Current or recent difficulties should be sought with both a general question such as, "Does your disease [i.e., the present illness] interfere with any part of your personal or sexual life?," and a specific inquiry into effects the patient may have noticed of **medications**. Medications and therapies may have a profound effect on a patient's sexual life and are probably underdiagnosed as etiologic agents in sexual disorders. For example, antihypertensives such as propranolol may induce male impotence. The patient may be reluctant to mention this side effect either because he does not associate it with the drug or because he does not wish to "displease" the physician who prescribed or advocates the medication.

VII. Medications and habits. This portion of the interview is devoted to discovering the names and dosages of all medicines presently or recently used by the patient. It also investigates smoking and drinking habits and the use of over-the-counter medications on a regular basis.

A. Medications. The name, dosage, and regimen of each drug the patient is using should be discussed. Any drugs that have been recently discontinued or used intermittently should be inquired about as well.

B. Habits. Tobacco smoking should be quantitated as should ethanol intake. Also ask about the use of recreational drugs at this point. In addition, habits that may be relevant physiologically should be sought, such as coffee and tea usage, over-the-counter analgesics (aspirin, acetaminophen), laxatives, birth control pills, sleeping medication, and diet pills.

VIII. Review of systems. In this portion of the history interview, all organ systems not already discussed during the present illness are systematically reviewed. The Review of Systems (ROS) is the last portion of the interview, and it serves three purposes: (a) to provide a thorough search for further as yet undiscovered disease processes, (b) to remind the patient of possible as yet unmentioned symptoms or difficulties he or she may be experiencing, and (c) to remind the physician in a logical manner of points of inquiry that may have been inadvertently omitted. The ROS purposely contains a minor amount of redundancy in the interest of thoroughness and is a final methodic inquiry prior to the physical examination. The topics to be reviewed for each organ system are outlined in Table 1-3. The table contains a master list of the topics in the ROS in the left column and selected clinical points of emphasis in the right column. Performance of the ROS and usage of the ROS table are further discussed in Part B.

XI. Conclusion of the history. After the Review of Systems, the physician concludes the history by offering the patient an opportunity to question or comment with a question such as, "Is there anything else you would like to discuss before I examine you?."

Table 1-3. Review of systems

System	Master list	Clinical points
Constitutional	Weight change	Recent change important.
	Anorexia	Acute or chronic?
	Fatigue	
	Weakness	
	Fever	Pattern (intermittent, remittent, sustained, or relapsing)? How documented?
	Sweats	Night? Drenching or mild? Frequency?
	Chills	Goose bumps vs. shaking (rigors)?
	Insomnia	Acute or chronic? When during night?
	Irritability	
Integument	Rashes	Local or generalized? Characterize.
	Itching	Diffuse?
	H/O skin trouble	Occupational? Allergic?
	Sores that do not heal	Squamous cell carcinoma? Poor diet? Drugs (e.g., steroids)?
	Bruising	Recent change?
	Bleeding disorders?	FHx?
Head	Headaches	
	Loss of consciousness	Cardiovascular vs. neurologic? Hx crucial.
	Seizures	Focal vs. general? Motor vs. absence?
	H/O trauma	When? Sequelae?
Eyes	Vision	Recent change? Glasses?
	Date last eye exam	
	FHx of glaucoma	Glaucoma often asymptomatic; hereditary with high penetration.
	Photophobia	Meningeal irritation?
	Pain	
	Redness	
	Irritation	

Table 1-3 (Continued)

System	Master list	Clinical points
	Excessive tearing	
	Diplopia	
	Scotomata	
Ears	Hearing	Recent change?
	Discharge or pain	H/O otitis? Trauma?
	Vertigo	Sensation of movement (vertigo) vs. dizziness.
	Tinnitus	Drug-related (aspirin)?
Respiratory Upper	Frequent colds	
	Sinus trouble	
	Postnasal drip	
	Nosebleeds (epistaxis)	Trauma? Other bleeding problems?
	Obstruction	Snoring history?
Lower	Cough	Chronic? A.M.? Productive? Recent change? Smoking history?
	Sore throats	
	Sputum	Amount? Color? Character? Recent change?
	Shortness of breath	Dyspnea? Rest or exertional? Accompanying chest discomfort?
	Wheezing	Seasonal? Episodic? Known allergens?
	Hemoptysis	Oral (e.g., dental) vs. pulmonary (e.g., bronchitis) vs. cardiac (e.g., mitral stenosis). Frank blood vs. tinged sputum vs. pink sputum?
	H/O chest illness	TB exposure? Bronchitis? Emphysema? Asthma? Pneumonia(s)?
	H/O smoking	Quantitate no. of pack-years. If "no," quit recently?
Lymphoreticular	Increased node size	Tender vs. painless? Location? Reactive (infections? systemic disease? drug?) vs. infiltrative? How first noticed? Any AIDS risk factors?
Breasts	Swelling	Unilateral or bilateral? Associated changes? Tender?
	Lumps	Recent change? transient or persistent? Menstrually related?
	Pain	Unilateral or bilateral? Trauma?
	Discharge	Milk (galactorrhea) vs. serous vs. blood? Unilateral or bilateral?
	Do you do self-exam?	Be able to teach during PE.
Cardiovascular	Chest pain or discomfort	Major DDx: CV vs. GI vs. musculoskeletal.

Table 1-3 (Continued)

System	Master list	Clinical points
	Palpitations	If ⊕, ask patient to tap out rate and rhythm. Syncope history? Any particular time when increased?
	Blood pressure	Usual range? H/O ↑ or ↓? FHx? Medications?
	Shortness of breath	Paroxysmal nocturnal dyspnea (PND)? Exercise tolerance? Exertion induced?
	Orthopnea	No. of pillows? If ⊕, what happens when patient reclines without pillows?
	Edema	Generalized (e.g., CHF, liver disease, nephrotic syndrome) or localized?
	Leg pain, cramps	Relieved by rest (intermittent claudication) vs. unremitting or night time (muscular)?
	Other cardiac Hx	H/O murmur(s), thrombophlebitis, "blood clots," varicose veins, "large" heart. Other cardiac medications? Rheumatic fever?
	Risk factors	Smoking, hypertension, hypercholesterolemia, DM, gout, obesity, FHx?
	Nocturia	Quantitate.
Gastrointestinal	Dentures, problems with teeth, oral lesions	Bleeding gums, ulcers, sores.
	Dysphagia	Where? (have patient point and describe): invariably heralds organic disease.
	Heartburn (pyrosis)	How do they find relief?
	Other symptoms of indigestion	Bloating, belching, flatulence; food-related Hx critical.
	Nausea	Relation to food, H/O GI disease and surgery, associated symptoms and signs.
	Vomiting	All medication, H/O weight loss, psychosocial factors.
	Hematemesis	Color? H/O ulcer disease? H/O gastritis? (lesion usually proximal to ligament of Treitz)
	Abdominal pain, discomfort	Hx critical. Acute vs. chronic? GI vs. reproductive?
	Food intolerance	Mild products? Gluten-containing, fried or fatty foods? H/O gall bladder disease?
	H/O GI disease	Hepatitis, ulcer disease, gall bladder disease, pancreatitis, diverticulitis, hemorrhoids?
	Hematochezia	Often suggests distal lesion; hemorrhoids most common but R/O neoplastic.

Table 1-3 (Continued)

System	Master list	Clinical points
	Jaundice	FHx? Viral-drug exposure? Associated Sx and/or signs?
	Change in stool	Color, consistency, unusual odor, oiliness, mucus? Caliber?
	Diarrhea	Acute vs. chronic? Infectious, drug or laxative? Dietary, inflammatory?
	Constipation	Mechanical vs. systemic illness vs. drug-induced vs. neurologic?
Genitourinary		
Urinary	Polyuria	Recent change? (Common causes: DM, renal disease, iatrogenic.)
	Dysuria	UTI "triad" (dysuria, frequency, urgency), but R/O genital disease.
	Hematuria	Painless (primary renal disease) vs. painful (e.g., UTI, stones, renal infarct)?
	Nocturia	How often? Recent change?
	Hesitancy	In older men along with ↓ stream, dripping, incontinence, C/W prostatic hypertrophy. Medications?
	Other renal Hx	UTIs? Stones or gravel in urine? Flank pain?
	Testicular swelling	Painful vs. painless?
Menstrual	Menarche	Cycle length, regularity, duration and amount of bleeding.
	Amenorrhea	Primary vs. secondary?
	Menorrhagia (profuse)	
	Metrorrhagia (intermenstrual)	
	Date last period	
	Date last pap smear	
	Pregnancies	Gravida ___ Para ___ Abortions ___ Miscarriages ___
	Vaginal discharge	H/O vaginal infections? Itching?
Venereal disease	H/O VD	If ⊕, what Rx did patient receive?
	H/O penile discharge	
	H/O chancre	
Sexual history		Must be tailored to patient (see Part B, **VI. C**). AIDS risk?
Musculoskeletal		
Joints	Pain	Location? Acute vs. chronic? H/O trauma? H/O previous infection? Present medication? FHx? H/O gout? Morning vs. evening stiffness?

Table 1-3 (Continued)

System	Master list	Clinical points
General	Weakness	
	Cramping	
	H/O back difficulties	Low back strain, osteoar-thritis, and disc disease are common causes.
	H/O trauma, fracture	
	H/O endocrine disease	
	Diabetic symptoms	Weight change, polyuria, polyphagia, polydipsia.
	Thyroid symptoms	Goiter, heat-cold intolerance, change in metabolic rate.
	Change in head, glove, shoe size	Acromegaly; change in head size only may be c/w Paget's disease.
Nervous system	Neuro difficulties in past	H/O stroke, seizures, childhood illness.
Motor	Atrophy	Location, time course, change in normal function.
	Weakness	Location, asymmetries? (Quantitate.)
	Involuntary movements	Tremor, fasciculations, seizure Hx.
Sensory	Anesthesia	Recent burns?
	Paresthesia	
	Hyperesthesia	
Mental status	Cortical function change	Memory changed? Reading, writing changed?

Note: *At the end of the ROS, it is useful to ask two questions:* (1) "Is there anything else bothering you?" (2) "Is there anything you would like to bring up or ask about before I give you a physical exam?"

B   **Practical Points Concerning the
                                          Patient Interview**

I. Introduction: Before the interview

A. Patient's chart. The patient's medical record is still known as the *chart* in many institutions, a holdover from the days when all information was recorded on a chart at the foot of the bed.

You will often be assigned a patient who has accumulated a substantial chart from previous admissions that includes recent notes concerning the present admission. Should you read the chart before seeing the patient, and if so, how much?

1. In general, it is not a good idea to read the information concerning the **present** admission, especially when first learning how to interview and take a history.

2. There is nothing wrong with having knowledge of previous admissions or problems, provided that the HPI is respected and faithfully taken. The present admission may be for new disease processes; it may also concern new nuances of previous problems. Being forearmed with some knowledge of the patient's prior problems may be an advantage prompting further insightful questions during your interview.

3. The chart that has accumulated during this admission may be especially useful after you have finished your HPI and physical exam. Interact with it

---

In taking a history from a patient in the hospital, *always sit down in a chair at the bedside*. Taking the history standing up gives the patient the impression that you are in a hurry. It takes no more time and the patient is more at ease if you sit while taking the history.
Eugene Braunwald, M.D.

In *taking a history which involves repeated episodes* (e.g., eating, pain, colds), always start with the most recent episode and get the precise details concerning it, then work backward. Never ask general questions about all episodes.
Donald N. Medearis, Jr., M.D.

Never argue with patients. The upset patient usually has a hidden problem . . . you, his doctor, are simply the target at the time. Stay loose, and "be slow to anger, and abounding in kindness," but stand your ground if the patient appears to be pushing you around, or tries to take charge of his own treatment.
Thomas B. Fitzpatrick, M.D.

The complaint I hear most often about doctors is that they will not talk to their patients adequately. A friendly and sincere interest in a patient's problem breaks the ice. Keep your appearance such that a patient will trust you. ("If he doesn't button up his shirt, how will he sew up my head?") Explain every move of the physical examination before it is done. Be courteous, respectful, and confidential. Show continued interest while in contact with the patient. Reappear frequently and at predictable times. Be reachable.
John Shillito, Jr., M.D.

as a way to compare your understanding of the patient's story, as well as your physical findings, to those of more experienced physicians.

4. Despite (1) above, as you become more comfortable with interviewing and begin to do admissions, you will realize that the chart can be a very useful way to gain a rapid introduction to a patient's case. Do not assume that something has been "unfairly provided"—the work-up is not an exam. Similarly, realize that your responsibilities as an interviewer and as a care-giver are not lessened by the chart and other persons' input into the patient's care.

B. **Approaching the patient.** Although the patient in a teaching hospital generally knows that he or she may be seen by a medical student, you are still obligated to explain your status. This is usually done by introducing yourself and saying, for instance, "Hello, Mr. Jones. I'm Ted Smith, the medical student who will be working with Dr. Thomas on your case." Remember, however, that the patient is confined to the hospital with a threatening and uncomfortable experience and that your visit may be sensed as an irrelevant intrusion. If you sense hostility it may be prudent to have the patient's main doctor introduce you as a member of the team. Adamant refusal is uncommon, and if it occurs often it may be time to reevaluate your approach.

C. When first learning to interview, you will occasionally be sent to interview a patient who is **clearly too ill** to be subjected to yet another history and physical exam. At such times it becomes necessary to take the initiative and after a brief visit with the patient, return to your preceptor, explain the situation, and find a new patient to interview.

D. **Do not introduce yourself as a doctor.** If the patient wishes, he or she may call you "Dr. Smith" after you have explained your medical student status, but it is misleading and unwise legally to introduce yourself as a physician. Patients will respect you for being a medical student; the discomfort associated with stating that fact often is a part of the natural insecurity involved with learning to be on the wards. Other physicians will not uncommonly introduce you as a doctor. In general, that moment is not the time to redefine your position. However, you may explain to the patient at a later time that you are in fact a medical student.

E. **Greeting the patient** when first entering the room begins with an introduction followed by a brief conversation that is not medical but rather an exchange of pleasantries, an attempt to find out how the patient is feeling in general without yet pursuing the specific. The point here is to help both you and the patient feel a bit more at ease before beginning with the introductory information and questions about the chief complaint.

F. It is a good idea to take a **clipboard** with scratch paper into the interview so that you can jot down brief notes during the HPI, record information that will be difficult to remember, and note points to which you wish to return.

In the beginning you will find yourself writing down much of what is said. Try not to devote yourself more to the notes than to the patient. You will find brief notes especially useful when inquiring about the past medical history, the family history, medications and habits, and the review of systems.

G. As was mentioned earlier, **introductory information** is often obtained from the chart. The addressograph plate that is made for each patient contains the patient's name and identifying data. You may wish to stamp the top of your note sheet or a memo card for each patient you interview (see Chap. 10).

II. Chief complaint (CC) and its duration

A. Many clinicians recommend using the **patient's own words** to describe the chief complaint in the write-up. Now is the time to record just what is said in response to your questions about why the patient has come to the hospital.

B. **The chief complaint may not be immediately obvious** since patients will not uncommonly complain of several things. Listen for a minute and try to pinpoint or determine the main problem that caused the patient to seek medical attention. **Taking a stance** is central to developing clinical skill. The learning process in medicine is based on decision-making and the acquisition of knowledge and confidence. Drawing conclusions that prove to be erroneous and emphasizing inappropriate data are expected consequences of learning to organize a case, and thoughtful mistakes will be respected. Therefore, choose a chief complaint and record other complaints to be placed after the HPI in your write-up (see Chap. 10).

C. Be sure to ask about and consider the **duration** of the chief complaint, which is a very useful clue in constructing the differential diagnosis during the next stages of your work-up, the history of the present illness.

D. Realize that the **chief complaint** may be very different from what you subsequently consider to be the patient's **most serious problem.** When a patient with a history of leukemia enters with a mouth ulcer, you may be more concerned about a possible relapse, but the chief complaint remains "my mouth is very sore."

III. History of the present illness

A. As a student, your primary goal in taking the HPI should be to get the patient to relate for you a clear **sequence of the events** that led the patient to seek medical attention. This interview should be both **specific** and **quantitative** ("I felt the pain all across my chest and down my left arm." "I can only walk half a block before I get tired."). To obtain this sort of HPI, you will have to use a combination of careful listening and skillful, goal-oriented questioning.

B. At first, when the interviewing process seems overwhelming, and later, when time is precious, it is easy to be too tired or harried to **listen well.** We cannot overemphasize that respect for and attention to the patient's story are central to any thoughtful work-up. Failure to listen to the patient's story and then react to it with refining questions is perhaps the most frequent difficulty of the beginning clinician. Do not allow the history to drown in concerns about the flood of further diagnostic steps (physical exam, lab work) that it rightfully sets in motion.

Let the patient do as much explaining as possible without interrupting. Interject to clarify and prompt, but avoid leading questions. Give your patient several uninterrupted minutes before you delve into a dissection of the symptoms or attempt to order the events.

Also, be wary of patient's use of **medical jargon;** ask about symptoms, not about diagnostic phrases that may be offered by the patient.

C. There are specific **techniques in interviewing** that will help in encouraging and maintaining the flow of information. Basically, the interviewer can follow the patient's own leads by using these techniques, which include facilitation, reflection, clarification, responding with empathy, interpretation, and occasionally confrontation. We recommend the discussion in Bates [3]; another excellent source book for the beginning interviewer is Morgan and Engel [23].

D. In your mind, try to **organize the evolving story around calendar dates and clock times.** Realize that your first clue in this regard was the duration of the chief complaint. The history (and its subsequent write-up) are built on a chronologic foundation. If you become clear about the time course of the patient's problems, two things result. First, the case will be logically organized for yourself and later for your readers. Second, you will have further insight into the tempo of the disease, one of the cornerstones of diagnosis.

E. **Symptom analysis** was explained in detail in part A of this chapter. The scheme for symptom analysis in Table 1-2 is thorough and worth learning, but a mnemonic device to use when considering a symptom can be useful. Such a mnemonic (illustrated for the attributes of the symptom "pain") is presented in DeGowin and DeGowin [6]. The mnemonic is **PQRST:**

Provocative-palliative factors
Quality of the pain
Region of the pain
Severity of the pain
Temporal characteristics

F. Do not be afraid to **requestion** the patient about points that are unclear or that seem crucial to your understanding of the case. People forget to mention things and may be reminded of them the second time, or they may dismiss what seems unimportant to them. Generally, the first time you ask a question you will take an open-ended stance ("Did you have any blood in your urine?"). The second time you can be more direct ("And you have seen blood in your urine only once?").

G. It is useful to stop and **summarize** your understanding of the details the patient has recounted at select points during the interview and especially *as you conclude the HPI* and get ready to begin the past medical history. Say something such as, "Let me see if I have this straight now," and then pause and summarize the patient's HPI, as you understood it, aloud to him or her. This encourages you to construct the story in a concise, uncluttered form and allows the patient to edit out errors and supplement areas of omission.

Once you become good at the summarizing process, the write-up of the HPI will be a lot easier.

H. At some point during the interview you should ask directly **what the patient thinks is wrong** and what features of the symptoms are causing the most worry. If the patient's fears are not addressed, the patient will undoubtedly leave the interview with some measure of anxiety. In addition, you may gain a new insight into the nature of the problem.

IV. Past medical history

A. The best way to **begin the PMH** is to ask a question such as, "Now, have you had any other medical problems or illnesses besides what we just discussed?" Often patients, especially older ones, will have trouble recalling their earlier medical history and will forget to mention illnesses that are chronic and treated, such as diabetes. It may help to prompt them with questions about prior admissions, but it will often be necessary to refer to the old chart. Turn to the PMH section of the typed discharge summary from the previous admission, which provides a good place to begin constructing a list of "other medical problems."

B. Although other medical problems may have been brought up during the discussion of the present illness, **specific discussion of each problem** identified takes place now. Make a quick note of various diagnoses or problems poorly remembered by the patient and you can consult the chart for further details.

C. Patients commonly deny any **allergies**. There are instances when more specific questions are important. For instance, if you think antibiotics may be important in a patient's management, you might ask, "Have you ever had penicillin before?" Because penicillin or penicillin derivatives are extremely useful and allergic reactions are their biggest disadvantage, a specific inquiry is merited. Similarly, patients admitted for cardiac catheterization should be asked about past allergic reactions to shellfish.

It is also important to distinguish between drug allergies and allergies to environmental factors. You need to clarify whether you are asking about drugs or about asthma, as the case may be.

D. **Childhood illnesses** may be sought with a general question such as, "Were you ever seriously ill as a child?" If the patient gives a positive response it is important to determine how the diagnosis was made, how long the problem lasted, and whether there were any sequelae. Patients who claim to have had rheumatic fever, for instance, should be asked whether they have had a rash (erythema marginatum), painful joints, uncontrolled movements especially of their hands (Syndenham's chorea, or "St. Vitus' dance"), or any evidence of heart difficulties since that time.

E. In gathering information about previous hospitalizations a question that seeks a specific history of **prior surgery** often will jog the patient's memory.

V. Family history

A. Record the information given about the patient's family by constructing a quick, simple **pedigree diagram.** Males are represented with squares, females with circles. Living relatives' ages are recorded within the circles or squares, deceased relatives' circles or squares are colored in. Specific diseases are pencilled in next to the appropriate symbol for the relative with the history of that disease. The patient is included on the diagram and identified with a bold arrow. For a sample diagram, see the FHx portion of the sample write-up in Chap. 10.

B. Do not forget to ask whether any **family members** have symptoms or diseases related to those described by the patient in the present illness.

VI. Psychosocial history

A. The psychosocial history is perhaps the most variable portion of the medical history. It is the section of the interview that focuses on the patient's lifestyle, homelife, work, and anxieties, in an effort to develop a more complete idea of the patient as a person. Because you may have gained some of this information in a less formal manner during the course of your conversation, the time required for the psychosocial history varies. **The key insights to gain relate to the ways in which the patient's daily life may interact with his or her disease, both physiologically and psychologically.** A sedentary 70-year-old man with occasional back pain when bending will have very different therapeutic needs than an active 40-year-old with similar pain.

B. As in other portions of the history, **general, open-ended questions** are good ways to initiate a discussion. For example, "How do you spend a typical day?" or "Tell me about your life at home." may be a useful starting point. In asking about occupation, both general questions ("What sort of work have you done in your life?") and directed ones ("Have you ever worked in a place where you were exposed to fumes or chemicals?") may be appropriate.

C. In beginning the **sexual history,** the ease with which the patient is able to discuss his or her private life will be related to your own ease in discussing and asking about sexual matters. One good beginning question is, "Are you satisfied with your sexual life?" It then becomes *crucial* to pay attention to both verbal and nonverbal responses by the patient. Generally you will be able to sense whether or not people have more to say on the subject; if so, you can facilitate the discussion by being receptive and understanding. On the other hand, a patient who is comfortable with his or her sexual life will usually make that fact clear.

D. It is well worth reading a more thorough discussion concerning the sexual history, such as that found in Bates [3] or in Morgan and Engel [23].

VII. Medications and habits

A. As the patient lists **medications** out loud, jot down each entry on a note pad in three columns. For example:

Drug name	Dose	Regimen
propranolol	40 mg	bid

B. If a patient cannot remember the name of a medicine, ask for a description of the medicine and the reason for its use; you can later describe it to a more experienced clinician who will probably be able to identify the drug. Also, you can ask patients if they have brought along their pill bottles, on which the information you seek is conveniently typed.

C. Quantitate carefully your patient's **alcohol intake.** Use measures that are familiar (e.g., number of six-packs, number of martinis, quarts of vodka). Realize that patients may underestimate (some clinicians mentally double or triple their patients' estimates in thinking about consumption) but record what the patient states to be used in your write-up later.

    D. Quantitate **smoking** in pack-years (1 pack-year equals 1 pack per day for 1 year). For example, a patient who smoked 2 packs per day for 3 years but cut back to 1 pack every other day for the past 2 years has a 7 pack-year history.

VIII. Review of systems

    A. Do this portion of the history **quickly and efficiently.** Explain to patients that you must ask a long series of questions, but that they may simply answer "no" after each question that does not apply to them. If there are review of systems questions that do apply, you must suspend the rapid style just described and analyze the positive finding in the same way as any symptom (see **III. E** and Part A, **III. A**).

    B. Avoid unnecessary repetition. Although some redundancy will occur as explained earlier, it is not necessary to review the organ system(s) you covered during the HPI interview unless there is a particular point you want to clarify.

    C. Recent changes are the most important points to glean from the ROS. Has the patient's exercise tolerance decreased recently or has she been fatigued after climbing stairs for several years? Did the patient begin to have night sweats this year or has he always had them in summertime? Patients may bring up several issues in one or more organ systems. It takes experience to know which complaints are more significant but those that have not appeared or changed recently will usually assume a lower place on your list of priorities as you organize the case.

    D. If a patient points to a lesion during the ROS, state that you will return to it while doing the physical exam, and continue your questioning.

    E. Table 1-3 contains a master list of ROS topics. The clinical points listed in the right-hand column are a collection of ideas meant to stimulate further thought on your part. They are not necessarily points to explore with each patient.

IX. Concluding the history. The patient is offered a chance for questions at the end of the history. Realize that you can always return to history questions later during the physical exam, or on a later visit. The sequence explained in this chapter is designed to help retrieve most of the important data necessary for working up a patient's case and to begin constructing a logical framework for considering the case. The next step in that framework is the physical examination.

If a *positive systems review* includes itching of the teeth, the sedimentation rate will probably be within the normal range.

K. Frank Austen, M.D.

The symptom *fatigue* is often hard to elicit by history. It is a negative symptom. It is a lack of energy.

Lewis Dexter, M.D.

There are three issues which must be understood and addressed in *the care of adolescent–young adult patients*. First, the history must be given by the patient alone. Parents may, of course, make their contribution, but not initially. Second, the physical examination is not complete unless the sexual maturation stage is noted and recorded. Third, the patient must be informed at the close of the evaluation what the diagnostic possibilities are, what tests and studies are necessary and why, and what treatment is planned, giving the responsibility to the patient, not the parents, for carrying out the therapy. Following these simple guidelines will open up the opportunity for you to talk about and counsel in the more sensitive areas of behavior, sexuality, education, career decisions, drugs, and alcohol. Care for your adolescent patients—don't delegate and triage!

Robert P. Masland, Jr., M.D.

2

The Physical Examination

The physical examination follows and complements the history in the sequence of the work-up. Each patient is examined systematically in a generally **head-to-toe** sequence to ensure thoroughness and to screen for abnormalities. In addition, a search for **specific** physical findings suggested by the interview occurs during this systematic exam: the history serves to focus and provide emphasis to the physical examination.

Part A of this chapter is an annotated outline of the physical examination presented telegraphically to allow bedside use. The right-hand column is an introduction to the correlation of physical findings with diagnostic significance. It contains comments on exam procedure and on positive and normal findings. Its goal is not to explain how to do the exam, which is carefully detailed in the recommended physical diagnosis textbooks [3, 6], but rather to answer some questions and address some frequent concerns that emerge during the specific exam sequence.

Part B of this chapter contains some practical advice concerning the physical exam addressed to the student who is inexperienced in physical diagnosis. It is followed by two appendices that present clinically relevant information:

Appendix 2-1: A summary of 15 common diagnostic signs used in physical diagnosis and description.

Appendix 2-2: Several annotated surface anatomy charts that will aid the student in correlating physical findings with organ involvement.

Infants and children are the most precious possessions that any parent has, and should be treated as such by the attending physician. They do have a first name and gender, and these should be used personally during history-taking. Most of us find all children attractive, and we ought not to be reluctant in sharing that feeling with the parent. The physical examination should be carried out by first attempting to interact with the child, then by doing a physical exam, proceeding with the least invasive things first, and the most disturbing events to the child (i.e., examination of ears and throat) at the end. Remember that the examining table was made for the convenience of the physician, and that the mother's lap and arms are the most comforting and secure areas for older infants and toddlers.

William Berenberg, M.D.

When you meet a patient, first decide if he is moving toward you or away, approaching or retreating. Sound clinical work must be done at the right distance. Patients in retreat may need to be approached and their experience shared, narrowing the distance. Patients moving in are often best not encouraged, reassured, or too much welcomed; they need a little more distance.

Leston L. Havens, M.D.

A   **Annotated Outline of the Physical Examination**

The following two-column chart is organized to outline a methodic approach to the physical examination. The order presented in the left-hand column is based on an anatomic, head-to-toe approach that is commonly employed by physicians. This column may be regarded as a checklist that will direct the examiner and enable him or her, with experience, to run smoothly through the physical exam.

The right-hand column is meant to be an introduction to the correlation of physical findings with diagnostic significance. This column contains comments on exam procedure and positive and normal findings. As explained earlier, its goal is not to explain details of the actual procedure but rather to address some common questions and concerns that emerge during the specific exam sequence.

I. General body habitus

  A. State of health and nourishment

  B. Obvious distress or affect problems

  C. Apparent age and vigor

  D. Grooming and expression

  E. State of consciousness

> Physical exam and mental status exam actually begin here; note speech patterns, lethargy, stupor, coma, intoxication, or anything else that will affect interpretation of the rest of the physical examination.

II. Vital signs and measurements

  A. Height and weight

> Weight is useful for following nutritional status and fluid balance. Height and weight are especially important in outpatient and pediatric exams; they are often recorded by the nurse when the patient is first admitted.

  B. Oral or rectal temperature

> Fever means infection until proved otherwise. Normal oral temperature fluctuates diurnally between 35.8°C (96.4°F) and 37.3°C (99.1°F).

  C. Pulse strength, rate, and rhythm

> Taking radial pulse is an unthreatening way to initiate physical contact. Note if irregularities are regularly irregular or irregularly irregular. Do beats drop occasionally? Sporadically? Note if the pulse is strong or weak. Compare to apical pulse during the cardiac exam.

  D. Blood pressure

> Hypertension is defined as >90 mm Hg diastolic and/or >140 mm Hg systolic. In patients with possible or known asthma, pericardial effusion, or emphysema, check for pulsus paradoxus (an inspiratory fall in systolic arterial pressure that exceeds 10 mm Hg). Recheck blood pressure if initial reading is elevated at some later point in the exam.

E. Respiratory rate and character

Note any respiratory patterns while taking the pulse. Do not announce intention to "count breaths," which may increase the patient's anxiety and alter normal breathing patterns. Consider the respiratory pattern again in the pulmonary and cardiovascular exams.

III. Hands. Temperature, color, appearance, nails, clubbing, nodes, contractures, degenerative changes

Compare general palm color to your own especially if considering anemia. Try to describe any degenerative changes seen. Note which interphalangeal joints are involved and which are spared. Note location of any nodules or swelling, or contractures; presence or absence of tenderness; and degree of motion remaining in the affected digits or limbs. Examine and describe for yourself changes in the **nails,** especially clubbing, deformities, or discolorations. For example:

clubbed nails   consistent with (c/w) numerous pulmonary diseases, cardiovascular diseases, and a large miscellaneous group.

spoon nails (koilonychia)   c/w iron deficiency or hypochromic anemias.

Mee's lines   c/w renal insufficiency, MI, infectious fevers, and poisonings, among others.

IV. Integument. Skin color, temperature, turgor, moisture, and lesions

Skin color: If suspicious of cyanosis, check for blue especially around mouth, nails, lips; look for the yellow of jaundice especially in the sclera. Decreased skin turgor is c/w dehydration or old age.

Skin lesions: Note type (macular, papular, nodular, eroded, ulcerated), shape (round, irregular), arrangement with respect to each other (discrete, clusters), and distribution on body (legs, trunk, face). Note especially lesions with irregular borders, heterogeneity of colors, and inflammatory regions. The majority of skin malignancies do not cause pruritis or pain. If a suspicious lesion is found, ask the patient: How long has it been present? Has it changed? Does it seem not to heal? (See also Colorplates E–I.)

Skin exam may be continued throughout the physical exam. Draw quick diagrams on your clipboard and quantitate when possible.

V. Head

A. Skull shape, scalp, lesions

B. Hair distribution

C. Characteristic facies

Characteristic facies include the edematous, myxedematous, Cushingoid, acromegalic, and Parkinsonian.

VI. Ears. Auditory canals, eardrums

Check for a light reflex and for fluid behind the eardrum.

The ear exam is especially important in the pediatric exam.

VII. Eyes

A. Eyelids, conjunctivae, and sclera

Look for xanthelasma, which suggest hypercholesterolemia. Note whether palpebral fissures are unequal as a clue to ptosis. Evert the lower lid and estimate the degree of "redness" of conjunctival vessels. Correlate this finding later with the patient's hematocrit to begin to screen for anemia. Note whether scleral yellowing is even or focal (even yellowing implies jaundice).

B. Extraocular movements

Actually part of neurologic exam, done now for convenience

Note: Other cranial nerves may be tested while examining the head and face.

C. Pupillary size

D. Direct and consensual pupillary reaction to light and accommodation

Anticholinergics cause dilated pupils. Opiate intoxication causes pinpoint pupils. Argyll-Robertson pupil (accommodation but no reaction) is c/w syphilis.

E. Visual fields

Visual fields are assessed quickly by confrontation method to examine the integrity of cranial nerve II and its connections.

F. Visual acuity

Ask patients what usual vision is; visual acuity may be quickly checked with a pocket-size Snellen chart.

G. Ocular pressure by gentle palpatation

Difference between left and right ocular pressure c/w glaucoma.

H. Ophthalmoscopic exam of fundi

Note opacities of the lens and fundoscopic abnormalities (arteriovenous nicking, hemorrhages, exudates, arteriolar narrowing); check for papilledema.

The fundoscopic exam is especially important in diseases with microvascular sequellae, such as hypertension and diabetes mellitus.

VIII. Nose. Septal position, nasal discharge, sinus tenderness, turbinate exam, airway patency

Sinusitis may be brought out by flexing neck and lowering head or by tapping over ethmoid, maxillary, and frontal sinuses. If it is suspected, ask the patient whether sinus difficulties have been a problem.

The most common cause of epistaxis is nose picking.

IX. Mouth and throat

A. Lip conditions, cheilosis, gum and mucous membrane condition

Check for mucosal lesions (petechiae, apthous ulcers, areas of induration). Gingival hypertrophy is c/w puberty, pregnancy, dilantin therapy, leukemia, gingivitis.

B. Tongue color and condition

An abnormally smooth, red tongue is c/w vitamin B_{12} or iron deficiency (atrophic glossitis). Familiarize yourself with the appearance of the common normal variations (geographic tongue, scrotal tongue).

Note any bleeding of the gums.

C. Dentition

Note the state of the teeth and whether any are missing.

D. Oropharynx

Note especially any unusual breath odor, hoarseness, lesions, or excessive salivation (ptyalism) or redness (injection).

X. Neck and axilla

A. Lymphadenopathy

Characterize cervical and axillary adenopathy: note number, location, tenderness or lack of tenderness, texture (rubbery vs. soft), and mobility. Recall that some "shotty" adenopathy is common, especially in inguinal area and in children.

B. Trachea position

Tracheal deviation may suggest a mass effect, pneumothorax, loss of lung volume, or fibrotic change.

C. Thyroid

Note thyroid size, mobility, and symmetry. It is often easier to see and feel the thyroid when the patient swallows (provide a cup of water). The thyroid exam may be repeated when standing behind the patient.

(MOVE TO BACK OF PATIENT)

XI. Back

A. Spinal column curvature and tenderness

Forward flexion of trunk may make scoliosis and kyphosis more obvious.

B. Costovertebral angle (CVA) tenderness

Extreme CVA tenderness is c/w acute kidney disease. Minor CVA tenderness is c/w low back pain of any etiology.

XII. Chest exam

A. Inspection

    1. Symmetry and shape of chest

Follow the sequence of inspection, palpation, percussion, and auscultation. Barrel chest is c/w obstructive lung disease (especially emphysema) and normal aging.

    2. Respiratory pattern

Note rate, rhythm, and regularity, and depth. Normal rate is 12–18 cycles/min for adults; it may be 35–40 in infants.

Resting shallow tachypnea is c/w restrictive lung disease. Hyperpnea is commonly c/w anxiety or exertion.

Rapid, deep Kussmaul breathing is seen in metabolic acidosis. Decreased respiratory rate is c/w a CNS respiratory depression.

Cheyne-Stokes breathing (alternating hypernea and apnea) is c/w normal sleep, heart failure, uremia, and CNS dysfunction.

B. Palpation

    1. Thoracic excursion

Note by inspection and palpation the presence or absence of symmetry and excursion of the thoracic wall. In trauma patients check for paradoxical inward buckling of chest during inspiration (flail chest).

C. Percussion

    1. Diaphragmatic descent

Normal descent is approximately 3–6 cm with full inspiration. Compare both sides and note any gross asymmetries in movement.

    2. Resonance

Compare percussion notes of right and left lung fields. Dullness is often caused by pleural thickening or consolidation.

Palpate for tactile fremitus if consolidation is suspected.

D. Auscultation

    1. Posterior chest

Compare the corresponding sites in right and left fields.

Check for presence of breath sounds at both bases and for adventitious sounds (crackles, wheezes, or rubs). Listen for egophony, whispered pectoriloquy, and fremitus when appropriate.

Airway deflation and pulmonary consolidation often lead to egophony, crackles, and/or increased fremitus. Bronchitis and asthma often cause crackles, wheezes, and an increased expiratory-inspiratory ratio.

(MOVE TO FRONT OF PATIENT)

2. Anterior chest

Always check apices of lungs; some diseases have primarily apical findings (e.g., TB).

XIII. Breast exam

A. Inspection

Have patient perform several maneuvers: arms at side, over head, pressed against hips.

Dimpling, contour asymmetry, venous prominence, redness, and nipple retraction may all be c/w breast cancer.

Draw diagrams indicating findings and specifying position with respect to the nipple.

(PATIENT LIES DOWN)

B. Palpation

Use a systematic manner of palpating. Note tenderness, nodularity, nipple discharge.

Nodules may be c/w fibrocystic breast disease, benign fibroadenomas, or carcinoma. Malignant lesions are typically firm, irregular, and neither well encapsulated nor mobile. Superficial signs of breast tissue retraction may be present. See sec. **III.C.6.**

XIV. Cardiovascular exam

A. Inspection

1. Jugular venous pulsation (JVP) level

Often best performed when patient's upper body is elevated with pillows at a 30-degree angle (see Fig. 3-1, p. 43).

The normal JVP is ≤8 cm. Increased JVP is c/w elevated right-sided pressures (consider elevated pulmonary pressures, right ventricular failure, tamponade or pericardial constriction or tricuspid valve disease).

2. Jugular contour of venous pulsation

Be sure you are inspecting the internal jugular system. Note A and V waves. The A wave is approximately synchronous with S_1, the V wave with S_2.

3. Point of maximal impulse (PMI), or apex beat

Search for the apex beat visually before palpating.

B. Palpation

1. Carotid pulse

See sec. **XV.**

2. Apex beat (PMI)

Note the position and character of the apex beat. An enlarged, prolonged, or displaced apex beat may indicate right or left ventricular hypertrophy or failure.

Note any other impulses or thrills, and whether they occur in systole or diastole.

C. Percussion

Try to determine extent of lateral heart border in patients in whom displacement of apex beat is noted.

D. Auscultation

1. Carotid arteries

2. First sound

S_1 created by closure of mitral, tricuspid valves.

3. Second sound

S_2 created by closure of aortic, pulmonic valves.

4. Third and fourth sounds

Check for any S_3 in diastole (created by rapid ventricular filling), which is found in normal children and young adults, pregnancy, heart failure, cases of increased cardiac output, and mitral and aortic insufficiency.

Check for any S_4 just preceding S_1 (created by the left atrium contracting into a stiffened left ventricle), which signifies pathology, especially left ventricular hypertrophy.

5. Other sounds

Including murmurs and rubs.

XV. Peripheral vascular pulses

A. Carotid, brachial, radial, femoral, popliteal, dorsalis pedis, and posterior tibial pulses

Weak pulses (pulsus parvus) c/w shock, heart failure, aortic stenosis. Increased pulse pressure c/w atherosclerosis, aortic regurgitation, high-output states. Delayed carotid upstroke c/w significant aortic stenosis (pulsus tardus). Pulsus alternans c/w LV failure. Right-left asymmetries in pulses suggest vascular diseases or shunts.

B. Bruits

Listen for bruits, which may be heard with atherosclerosis or aneurysms. Check the carotid and femoral arteries and listen in the abdomen for aorta and renal artery bruits.

XVI. Abdominal exam

A. Inspection

Draw a brief diagram on your clipboard to note data from the abdominal exam (see Chap. 10, Sample Write-Up).

Note any distention, scars, superficial lesions, or venous prominence. Venous prominence is seen with portal hypertension.

B. Auscultation

Note: Auscultation precedes palpation and percussion in the abdominal exam so that you can listen to the bowels while they are undisturbed.

Listen for bruits and bowel sounds; absence of bowel sounds for up to 1 minute may be normal.

C. Palpation

Note any rigidity, guarding, tenderness, organomegaly, or masses; watch the patient's face for change in expression as you palpate to help quantify degree of tenderness.

Note any kidney tenderness or enlargement. Palpate the liver edge for texture, contour, and tenderness. Remember that the spleen is usually not palpable in the normal adult.

D. Percussion

   1. Percussion note

Note character of percussion note (gas percusses with a hollow, tympanitic sound; fat, fluid, and underlying tissue percuss with dull sounds).

   2. Liver and spleen

Percuss for size of liver and spleen and define the extent to which they extend below the costal margin.

   3. Shifting dullness

In cases with possible ascites, check for dullness that shifts as patient changes position. Look also for a fluid wave.

XVII. Inguinal area

Check for inguinal adenopathy and for femoral pulses and bruits.

XVIII. Genital exam
Note: Pelvic and rectal exams are often performed at the end of the entire exam.

   A. Male

     1. Penis

Note the presence of any penile lesions or discharge (see Colorplate D, 7).

     2. Scrotum

Check for scrotal lesions and palpate spermatic cord.

     3. Testes

Check for testes bilaterally and evaluate shape and firmness.

     4. Hernia

Inspect for hernia; this may also be done later with patient standing.

   B. Female

See sec. **XXIII.**

XIX. Lower extremities

Note: This section of the physical examination is often used as a starting point for the musculoskeletal and neurologic examinations. Because these exams often involve returning to the upper extremities, they are outlined specifically below.

   A. Inspection

Note any skeletal and muscular deformities or asymmetries. Inspect for varicose veins. Examine the joints (see **B.1**). Look for color changes or decreased hair on the toes and feet.

   B. Palpation

     1. Joints

Check for tenderness, swelling, redness, and effusions.

2. Temperature

Check for the relative warmth of the feet and toes with the back of your hand as an indirect assessment of perfusion.

(PATIENT SITS UP AGAIN)

XX. Musculoskeletal exam

Note: This exam is one in which it is particularly important to focus on the symptomatic or suspicious areas pinpointed by the general screening questions and exam. For example, complete, quantitative range-of-motion testing is warranted only by specific history or findings consistent with musculoskeletal disease.

Ask again concerning joint or bone pain and have patient point to the specific area involved.

Listen throughout this exam for crepitations; inspect for joint swelling or deformities; and evaluate strength and range of motion.

A. Head and neck

If neck pain is present, it is important to check for upper motor neuron changes in the lower extremities and lower motor neuron changes in the upper extremities.

B. Shoulders

Pain may be generated from or referred to local structures.

C. Elbows

Warm, tender joints with subcutaneous nodules around the olecranon process suggest rheumatoid arthritis.

D. Hands and wrists

Palpable enlargement of bones in the hands is seen most commonly in degenerative joint disease (osteoarthritis).

Bilateral wrist swelling is seen in rheumatoid arthritis.

E. Spine

Always inspect contour carefully and test range of motion.

F. Hips

Pain and limitation of motion are common arthritic sequelae.

G. Knees

Note presence of *genu varum* (bowlegs) or *genu valgum* (knock-knees).

H. Feet and ankles

Gout commonly affects the metatarsophalangeal joint of the first (big) toe.

XXI. Neurologic exam (screening)

Note: Many patients do not receive a full neurologic exam but instead are given only a screening exam when no abnormality is suspected.

A. Sensory exam: pinprick, vibration sense, position sense, light touch

Check symmetric areas in right and left limbs; symmetric loss is c/w peripheral neuropathy.

If vibration sense is intact in the distal toes you need not proceed proximally.

B. Reflexes

Note any right-left asymmetries. Record the findings on a clipboard by drawing a stick figure (see Chap. 10, Sample Write-Up).

C. Biceps, triceps, brachioradialis, patella, Achilles tendon reflexes

Upper motor neuron lesions cause spasticity; lower motor neuron lesions cause flaccidity. Leg reflexes can be reinforced by isometric, opposed arm pulls.

D. Babinski reflex

Positive Babinski reflex is c/w upper motor neuron disease.

E. Mental status

Orientation is evaluated in every patient; a more complete mental status exam is conducted only in select instances.

F. Orientation to person, place, time

First lost is time orientation, then orientation to place, and then to person.

G. Appearance, behavior, speech patterns, tics, mood and affect, thought process and cognitive function

Depression hallmarks: helplessness, hopelessness, worthlessness. Important to ask about suicidal inclinations if there is any possibility.

Bizarre, paranoid thoughts c/w schizophrenic disorder.

If indicated, test proverb interpretation, calculating ability, serial 7s, long- and short-term memory.

H. Motor, coordination, gait, Romberg sign

Note: This portion of the neurologic exam overlaps with the musculoskeletal exam.

Check both cerebellar tests (finger-to-nose) and general coordination (heel and toe walking).

I. Cranial nerves

The cranial nerves that have not yet been tested are returned to (all may have been done early in the exam while examing the head and neck).

The cranial nerves I through XII are as follows:

Number	Name	Actions
I	Olfactory	Smell
II	Optic	Vision
III	Oculomotor	Most extra-ocular muscles; pupillary constriction

Number	Name	Actions
IV	Trochlear	Movement of eye down and in (superior oblique muscle)
V	Trigeminal	Sensory to face; motor to temporal and masseter
VI	Abducens	Lateral movement of eye (lateral rectus muscle)
VII	Facial	Motor to most of facial muscles; anterior tongue taste
VIII	Acoustic	Hearing and balance
IX	Glosso-pharyngeal	Pharynx-sensory and motor; posterior tongue taste
X	Vagus	Motor to palate, pharynx, larynx; sensory to pharynx and larynx
XI	Spinal accessory	Sterno-cleidomastoid and trapezius motor
XII	Hyperglossal	Motor to tongue

(PATIENT IS APPROPRIATELY POSITIONED AND DRAPED)

XXII. Rectal exam

A. Anal lesions, sphincter tone, stool color, male prostate size

Prostate exam is especially important in men over 50 years old.

The rectal exam is part of the pelvic exam in the female.

B. Guaiac test

Always check for occult blood with a guaiac test.

XXIII. Pelvic exam

A. External exam, labia, urethral orifice, introitus, perineum

Careful inspection for irritation, discharge, or lesions occurs here.

B. Speculum exam, cervix and os specimens (endocervical swab, cervical scrape, and vaginal pool), vaginal canal exam.

The pap smear and gonococcal cultures are taken here.

The vaginal canal may be inspected as the speculum is removed.

C. Bimanual exam, cervix, fornix, uterus, ovaries

D. Rectal exam

The rectal exam is often done with simultaneous placement of a finger in the vagina to palpate the interposed tissue. Change gloves before doing this exam to decrease the likelihood of spreading infection.

B   **Practical Points Concerning the
                                               Physical Examination**

I. Introduction: Before the examination

A. The physical examination is an art that is learned only by constant repetition. You will learn a great deal through careful study of one of the many available physical examination manuals, but the only way to get comfortable with the techniques of the exam is to practice.

B. Although there are many individual styles and methods of conducting the general screening exam, every good physician will choose one examination sequence and stick to it. Most people prefer to work in a generally head-to-foot order, with exceptions made as necessary for convenience and completeness. As each part of the body is examined, it is usually best to follow an orderly sequence of **inspection, palpation, percussion, and auscultation.** This routine will help ensure thoroughness, and also will aid in putting the patient at ease by minimizing the unexpected.

C. The best way to learn physical diagnosis is through **repeated proctoring** of your methods. An experienced clinician can show you how to hold your hands just so; it is always easier to demonstrate than to explain.

D. Think in advance about **what you expect to find** in any given part of the exam. What kind of peripheral neurologic exam might you expect of a long-term diabetic? Are there other physical exam findings that might help you to gauge the progress of the disease?

E. The physical examination should always be conducted and assessed in the context of the patient's clinical history. The range of what is normal varies from patient to patient, and physical findings cannot be gathered and interpreted in a vacuum.

It is often helpful to *examine the lymph nodes* in the neck, supraclavicular areas, and axillae with the patient *in both the sitting and supine positions*. Subtle changes in muscle tone and posture may make enlarged nodes more conspicuous in one or the other position.

In *palpating for an enlarged spleen* the examiner should first be sure that the patient is lying entirely flat. Students and house officers tend to be too forceful in palpating the left upper quadrant; the spleen is usually soft and mobile and is best felt with a gentle hand. Exerting firm pressure from below on the lower rib cage with the other hand will sometimes make it easier to palpate a spleen tip, which is otherwise difficult to feel.

Stephen H. Robinson, M.D.

The neurologist is quite properly preoccupied with *the extensor toe response* as indicative of pathology in the corticospinal system. On occasion it is difficult to evaluate. Perhaps this is particularly true in infants where the response of toe to plantar stimulation is often correctly described as equivocal (which, in fact, means normal). There is, however, an abnormal toe response to plantar stimulation in the newborn, which is identified by its majestic, i.e., slow, response and full great toe extension usually accompanied by more than usual flaring of the other toes. In older infants and children, the issue is complicated by the very natural tendency voluntarily to withdraw. Withdrawal is minimized by stimulation to the lateral aspect of the foot by a blunt object. No keys! In some cases the examiner's thumb as the stimulating object is useful although this will offend the neurological purist. The object is information, not ritual.

Charles F. Barlow, M.D.

II. General points concerning the examination

A. Do not be alarmed if during the first few weeks you try the complete exam it takes you much longer than expected; first concentrate on learning each subsection, then work on stringing all the parts together smoothly.

B. Do not be afraid to **repeat** parts of the exam if the findings are equivocal. Realize, however, that the diagnostic success of your exam depends on the cooperation of the patient, and it is tedious and uncomfortable to be poked and maneuvered for hours at a time. It is often useful to repeat parts of the physical exam after looking at the results of the physical diagnostic tests; a patient whose chest x-ray shows some lobar consolidation provides a good opportunity to fine tune your auscultatory abilities.

C. **Practice** your exam techniques when you are away from the bedside. Take the time to familiarize yourself with your equipment, so that you will not, for example, fumble around with an inside-out blood pressure cuff. Practice on other medical students in order to get a good idea of the normal range.

D. Realize that the physical exam provides a perfect opportunity to **requestion** the patient concerning ROS topics you may have forgotten or may be unclear about. It is often quite natural to introduce your next step with a general question concerning the organ system being examined (e.g., begin the otoscopic exam with, "So you've had no difficulties with ear aches or infections?").

E. Part A of this chapter provides a complete list of the various components of the physical exam. Each exam you do is **tailored to the patient** involved and directed by his or her problems. You will learn to run rapidly through the organ systems that you do not suspect to be involved and quickly decide whether findings are within normal limits. This takes practice but it is certainly possible to do a brief, general screening physical in 10 minutes once you are familiar and facile with the parts of the exam.

III. Specific points concerning the physical examination

A. There are numerous **signs** in clinical medicine, many of which are named for their discoverers. However, a small number of signs occur frequently enough to warrant learning from the start. These signs are listed in Appendix 2-1, which appears at the end of this chapter.

B. **Surface anatomy** becomes important in performing the physical examination and is therefore summarized in Appendix 2-2.

C. There are six traditionally difficult or **problematic sections** of the physical examination: the funduscopic exam, the cardiac exam, the neurologic exam, the rectal exam, the pelvic exam, and the breast exam. Each of these is discussed specifically below.

   1. The **funduscopic exam** is very difficult to master. Work first on getting the "red reflex." If you have a cat in the house, the cat eye is an excellent place to practice since the pupil remains relatively dilated. If you are around when a patient's eyes are pharmacologically dilated for some reason, ask to be permitted to examine his or her eyes as well.

   Once the red reflex is easy to elicit, concentrate on visualizing the disc and then tracing its perimeter. Dial up and down 1 or 2 diopters in each direction after you have visualized an edge of the disc and try to get a sense of how the disc relates to the retinal surface. Realize that the beautiful textbook pictures of fundi are generated with a special ophthalmoscope that allows visualization of much more of the fundus than your hand-held model.

   Finally, begin to follow the course of the vessels from the fundus outward into the four quadrants. Do not subject your patient to too long an exam; divide it into two parts if necessary. Note where veins and arteries cross; look for nicking and other abnormalities. The funduscopic exam takes months to learn and years to master. In some patients it is impossible to visualize the fundi without dilating their pupils. (Remember that the ophthalmologist usually insists on dilating a patient before performing an exam.)

2. The **cardiac exam** is made up of several parts. Of these, auscultation of the heart usually takes the longest time to master (except for analysis of the jugular venous pulse contours, which most physicians and some cardiologists never master). Because it is important and difficult, the cardiovascular examination is discussed in detail in Chapter 3.

3. The **neurologic exam** is made up of five main parts: the mental status, motor, sensory, cranial nerve, and reflex exams. Because a thorough neurologic exam has so many specific parts, however, confusion often results, largely because the neurologic exam is approached in such a shotgun manner during a typical physical exam sequence.

When it is warranted, consider performing on appropriate patients a neurologic exam separate from and in addition to the usual screening physical exam. If you are working up a patient with neurologic disease, do a brief general screening exam, and then a more complete neurologic exam (see Appendix A, p. 225). With the neurologic examination as your specific (and only) task, it is much easier to organize your thoughts and work-up.

Patients with unexplained neurologic abnormalities and evidence of infection may warrant a lumbar puncture as an emergency procedure. Some of the common organisms seen in the CSF of infected patients are shown in Colorplate D (1, 5, and 8).

4. The **rectal exam** is sometimes difficult simply because it is unpleasant for patient and physician; it is not hard to learn or execute, however. (It does take practice to learn how to palpate the prostate and judge its size and firmness, but this becomes much easier after 10 to 20 exams.)

Relax yourself and your patient, be firm and gentle, and be sure to guaiac the small bit of stool that is invariably on your glove after the exam. In men, especially older ones, practice defining the lobes of the prostate, assess its texture, and search for focal areas of induration. In women the rectal is part of the pelvic exam in many cases and is important especially when defining the extent of gynecologic tumor and for the stool guaiac.

Do not be tentative about the rectal; it is a brief exam and a very important one. On the other hand, when first learning you will often examine patients who have already had several rectals. It is prudent to check the chart ahead of time to see how many rectals have been done, and to defer the rectal if one has been performed that day.

5. The **pelvic exam** is often considered separately for two reasons: it requires a special set-up, and it is an examination that is extremely sensitive and personal.

A male should never perform a pelvic examination without a female chaperone (nurse or physician) present.

The exam is best learned by spending a concentrated period of time doing several pelvic examinations each day, e.g., by going on an obstetrics-gynecology rotation, or by arranging to work for several consecutive days in an outpatient gynecology clinic.

Traditionally, the most difficult part of the exam is the speculum insertion. The speculum exam should be observed several times and then practiced with special attention to the warming and moistening of the speculum before insertion, the angle at which the speculum is introduced, and the opening of the speculum after it is fully inserted.

6. The **breast exam.** Like the blood pressure measurement, the breast examination is one of the few parts of the physical exam that will frequently yield crucial information prompting major medical interventions in the entirely asymptomatic patient. Nearly one of ten American women will develop breast cancer, and every medical student should be familiar with its signs.

   a. **Inspection.** The patient should be disrobed to the waist and both breasts should be inspected concurrently to allow comparison. During the various positioning maneuvers listed in sec. **XIII** on p. 27, pay particular attention to symmetry between the left and right breasts. Though it is quite common for one breast to be somewhat larger than the other, the asymmetry should not include major differences in the appearance or texture of the skin or the nipples, nor should there be lumpy irregularities in the normally smooth breast contours.

   Local areas of erythema and swelling may be due to tumor, inflammation, or merely to tight clothing and should be carefully scrutinized. While breast cancer with lymphatic engorgement may produce only subtle changes (peau d'orange, best seen with a tangentially directed flashlight), direct skin invasion often produces an angry red cellulitic appearance that is unmistakable. Except in the nursing mother, any nipple discharge should be regarded as suspicious. Skin retraction is one of the most subtle findings in this part of the exam. It is often best appreciated in the "arms over head" and "hands against hips" maneuvers. A small, innocuous looking bulge in the upper outer quadrant that moves up into the axilla when the arms are raised is a classic early finding in breast carcinoma.

   b. **Palpation.** Though many different sequences of breast palpation are used, they are all thorough, systematic, and bimanual. One good technique for the novice involves starting at the nipple and following a clockwise spiral pattern around the breast and into the axilla. The fingertips are used alternately to compress and push the breast tissue toward the other hand. The palms of the hand are less sensitive and do not play a major role in this technique. If a suspicious area is felt, it is localized under the examiner's fingertips with the arms down. The arms are then slowly raised over the head to allow an assessment of mobility of the lesion.

   In addition to such a careful breast exam, it is critical to thoroughly investigate the possibility of associated lymphadenopathy in the axillary and supraclavicular regions in all patients.

   The axilla must be deeply palpated with the patient's arm draped across the chest to accomplish maximal relaxation of the pectoral muscles. Once again, asymmetry between the left and the right may be the only clue to an abnormal finding.

   c. **Recording the exam.** Accurate recording of the breast exam is absolutely crucial and may spare the patient unnecessary surgery at some point in the future. It is usually best to accompany a verbal description with diagrams and precise polar coordinates (e.g., "a 2-cm by 3-cm freely mobile mass located in the 3 o'clock position, 2.5 cm from the areolar edge"). For premenopausal patients, the exact position in the menstrual cycle at the time of the exam should also be noted.

   d. **Benign processes** including chronic cystic mastitis and fibroadenomas are common in the breast, and the vast majority of breast masses are not malignant. However, serial breast exams with mammographic correlation provide the best means of detecting this very common malignancy in its early stages.

Appendix 2-1 — Fifteen Common Diagnostic Signs

Babinski reflex   Dorsiflexion of the big toe after stimulation of the lateral sole; associated with pyramidal tract lesions.

Brudzinski's sign   Flexion of the hip and knee induced by flexion of the neck; associated with meningeal irritation.

Cheyne-Stokes respiration   Rhythmic cycles of deep and shallow respiration, often with apneic periods; associated with CNS respiratory center dysfunction.

Chvostek's sign   Facial muscle spasm induced by tapping on the facial nerve branches; associated with hypocalcemia.

Fluid wave   Transmission across the abdomen of a wave induced by snapping the abdomen; associated with ascites.

Hoffmann's sign   Flexion of the thumb and other fingers induced by snapping the nail of the index, middle, or ring finger; associated with pyramidal tract disease.

Homans' sign   Pain behind the knee induced by dorsiflexion of the foot; associated with peripheral vascular disease, especially venous thrombosis in the calf.

Kernig's sign   Inability to extend leg when sitting or lying with the thigh flexed on the abdomen; associated with meningeal irritation.

Kussmaul's respiration   Paroxysmal air hunger; associated with acidosis, especially diabetic ketoacidosis.

Kussmaul's sign   Distention of the jugular veins on inspiration; seen in constructive pericarditis and mediastinal tumor.

Levine sign   Clenching of the patient's fist over the sternum while describing chest discomfort; associated with angina.

McBurney's sign   Tenderness at McBurney's point (located two-thirds of the distance from the umbilicus to the anterior superior iliac spine); associated with appendicitis.

Obturator sign   Pain induced by pressure on the obturator foramen; associated with obturator nerve irritation, often as a result of appendicitis.

Psoas sign   Pain induced by hyperextension of the right thigh while lying on the left side; associated with appendicitis.

Romberg sign   Unsteadiness or falling when the eyes are closed and the feet are close together; associated with tabes dorsalis and labyrinthine disorders.

Appendix 2-2 | **Anatomy and Surface Anatomy Diagrams**

Note the relations of the internal organs in Figs. 2-1 and 2-2 to the spinal column landmarks on Fig. 2-3.

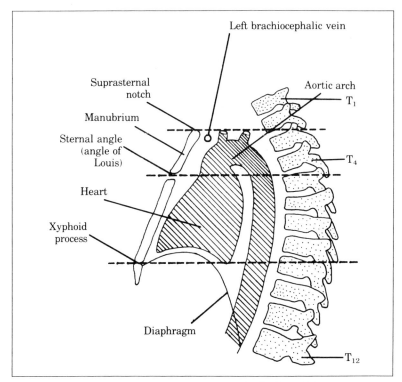

Fig. 2-1. The heart and aorta. (Redrawn from R. S. Snell, *Clinical Anatomy for Medical Students* [2nd ed.]. Boston: Little, Brown, 1981.)

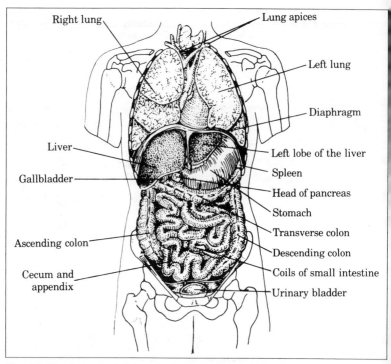

Fig. 2-2. The thorax and abdomen. (Redrawn from R. S. Snell, *Clinical Anatomy for Medical Students* [2nd ed.]. Boston: Little, Brown, 1981.)

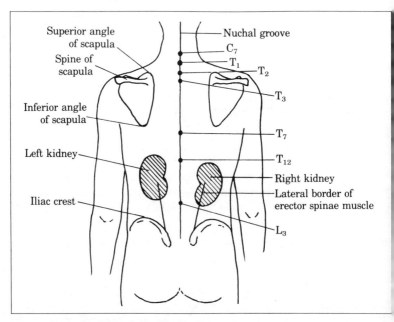

Fig. 2-3. The back. (Redrawn from R. S. Snell, *Clinical Anatomy for Medical Students* [2nd ed.]. Boston: Little, Brown, 1981.)

3

As the past two chapters have pointed out, the patient's symptoms and the history lend emphasis to the subsequent physical exam, helping to focus the examiner's search for physical findings.

It is important to realize that the general screening physical exam may be somewhat cursory. For example, if a patient has a problem that is neurologic in nature, a more in-depth neurologic exam would be in order. In fact, the exam pertinent to any organ system may be carried out in greater detail, and it is important to become familiar with the comprehensive exam of each organ system as well as with the general screening exam.

The cardiovascular (CV) exam is a case in point. There is a high prevalence of cardiovascular disease in our society, and a wealth of information can be gained from a detailed cardiovascular exam. For these reasons, and because most medical students feel that it is a somewhat intimidating exam, we have chosen to provide a brief chapter on the comprehensive cardiovascular exam. It is worthwhile to approach each case, especially when first learning the work-up, as a chance to practice the general screening exam, as well as the more detailed exam for the specific organ systems that seem to be involved in the patient's problem.

The first step in understanding and learning the cardiovascular exam (or the exam for any single organ system) is to outline the methodic approach to the system in question. Such an outline for the CV exam is presented in Table 3-1.

Part A of this chapter contains a short description of each topic outlined in Table 3-1. Part B provides some beginning tips about learning the CV exam as well as several reference tables concerning cardiovascular physical findings.

A   **Annotated Outline of the
                          Cardiovascular Examination**

I. Peripheral vascular findings

The purpose of approaching the cardiovascular system in a manner isolated from the remainder of the exam is in part to develop a mental picture of the functioning heart and its vessels. This process begins with measuring the blood pressure and peripheral pulses.

A. Blood pressure. The blood pressure is measured in both upper extremities, and then with the patient in two positions, **supine** and either **sitting or standing.** The degree of pulsus paradox is noted at this time as well.

The best advice that I have received about patient care was from the late Dr. Samuel A. Levine. His advice was simply, "Worry about your patient." By that he meant to urge us to think about individual patient problems and vexing diagnostic dilemmas, particularly when one is out of the hospital and away from the fray. Sometimes the best clinical ideas come when one is simply free associating while taking a walk and allowing one's mind to run free.

David G. Nathan, M.D.

Table 3-1. Organization of the cardiovascular exam

I. Peripheral vascular findings
   A. Blood pressure
   B. Peripheral pulses

II. Inspection
   A. Jugular venous pulse (JVP)
   B. Point of maximal impulse (PMI)
   C. Other precordial impulses

III. Palpation
   A. Carotid pulse contour
   B. Precordium
      1. Apex impulse
      2. Other precordial impulses or thrills

IV. Auscultation
   A. Vascular
      1. Carotids
      2. Other vessels
   B. Heart sounds
      1. First sound
      2. Second sound
      3. Third and fourth sounds
   C. Systolic sounds
   D. Diastolic sounds
   E. Extra cardiac sounds

B. Peripheral pulses. The radial pulse rate is taken with the patient both supine and either sitting or standing, and is correlated with the blood pressure measurements. The brachial, carotid, femoral, popliteal, posterior tibial, and dorsal pedal pulses are then systematically palpated and evaluated for their strength. The presence of bruits is sought in the carotid and femoral regions.

The carotid pulse is addressed more fully, as explained below.

II. Inspection

A. Jugular venous pulse. The jugular venous pulsation (JVP) is inspected in the patient's neck, as illustrated in Fig. 3-1. An attempt is made first to assess the height of the JVP column and then to examine the components of the pulsation for the A and V waves.

B. Point of maximal impulse. The point of maximal impulse (PMI) is the visual evidence for the apex beat of the heart or, in the case of a grossly abnormal precordium, is the area that is most obviously active during the cardiac cycle. It is sought by careful precordial inspection and most often can be found in the fifth intercostal space in the area of the midclavicular line.

C. Other precordial impulses. Further movements of the chest wall in response to the underlying activity of the heart are sought and noted.

III. Palpation

A. Carotid pulse contour. The carotid pulsation is palpated carefully for strength and contour. An attempt is made to correlate the carotid pulsation with the events of the cardiac cycle, and the pulse may be palpated during auscultation of the heart to help distinguish the heart sounds from one another.

B. Precordium

   1. Apex impulse. The apex beat (which usually generates the PMI) is next

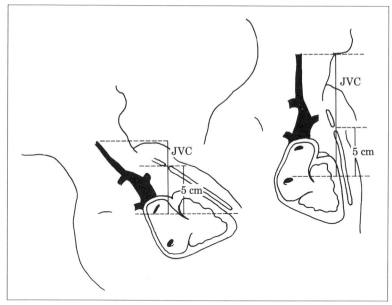

Fig. 3-1. The jugular venous pulse can be used as a manometer to measure right atrial pressure. Since the distance from the right atrium to the sternal notch is 5 cm, regardless of the patient's position (see above), right atrial pressure can be estimated by measuring the distance in centimeters from the sternal notch to the top of the jugular venous column (JVC). Then, right atrial pressure = 5 cm + JVC (cm). (Modified from R. Judge and G. Zuidema, *Methods of Clinical Examination: A Physiologic Approach*. Boston: Little, Brown, 1974.)

palpated, and the force and duration of the impulse are assessed.

2. **Other precordial impulses or thrills.** Further impulses are felt for at this point, both corresponding to and in addition to any that may have been seen during inspection of the precordium. **Thrills,** the tactile correlate of murmurs, are also sought now and again after auscultation.

IV. Auscultation

A. Vascular

1. **Carotids.** The main purpose of vascular auscultation is to search for the presence of underlying turbulence in the form of **bruits.** The carotids are also ausculted carefully for evidence of any murmurs radiating from the heart below. It is therefore often useful to return to the carotids when a murmur is appreciated and reevaluate the possibility of carotid radiation of the murmur.

2. **Other vessels.** A search for bruits is made in the femoral areas, and the abdomen is examined for the presence of renal artery bruits.

B. Heart sounds

1. **First sound.** The first heart sound (S_1), corresponding to the event of atrioventricular valve closure (first mitral, then tricuspid; see Fig. 3-2), is ausculted.

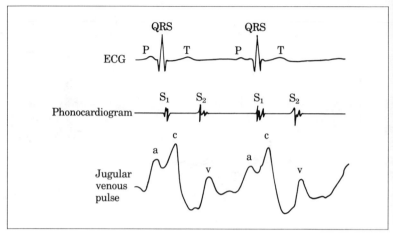

Fig. 3-2. Normal jugular venous pulse contour. Note the relationship between the first and second heart sounds, and the waves of the jugular venous pulse. Note also that the a and c waves are seen as one wave when observing the JVP contour.

   2. Second sound. The second heart sound (S_2), usually made up of the aortic and pulmonic components corresponding to valve closure, is next examined (Fig. 3-2), and its change with respirations is noted.

   For both S_1 and S_2, the intensity of the sound and its timing in relation to the other sounds and events of the cardiac cycle are evaluated.

   3. Third and fourth heart sounds. The presence or absence of a third heart sound (S_3) in middiastole is sought, and its variation with respiration, if any, is noted. The fourth heart sound (S_4) is sought in a similar manner. It is heard just preceding the first heart sound.

C. Systolic sounds. The period of systole is identified and the presence of any murmurs, clicks, or other sounds is noted. Any systolic murmurs appreciated are examined for their **radiation, variation with respiration, quality, timing,** and **variation with maneuvers.** Clicks and other sounds are examined with respect to their timing and variation with respiration.

D. Diastolic sounds. The period of diastole is identified and, as explained for systole (**C**), examined for the presence of murmurs or other sounds. Any murmurs noted are similarly characterized with respect to the variables noted for systolic murmurs (**C**). Diastolic murmurs in particular are sought by positioning the patient; murmurs of **atrioventricular valve incompetence** are sought in the left lateral decubitus position, and those of **semilunar valve incompetence** with the patient sitting up, leaning forward, and at end-expiration.

E. Extracardiac sounds. Any sounds with no apparent relation to the cardiac cycle are noted as well.

B   **Practical Points Concerning the
                                                Cardiovascular Examination**

I. Peripheral vascular findings

A. Blood pressure. In the routine screening exam, you will have recorded the blood
pressure with the rest of the vital signs, or you may have simply taken it with the
vital signs from the nurse's admission notes on the patient.

A more thorough evaluation of blood pressure is appropriate as part of the CV
exam. Careful systolic and diastolic pressures are recorded. Take orthostatic
blood pressure and pulse measurements on patients with low systolic blood pressures, clinical evidence of hypovolemia, complaints of dizziness, or those who are
febrile or who may have autonomic dysfunction.

In a patient with abnormal blood pressure, it is prudent to check the pressure in
the other arm at least once to help exclude the presence of aortic coarctation,
and it is also helpful to recheck an elevated pressure later in your exam since the
initial part of the physical exam may create enough anxiety to elevate the
patient's blood pressure.

Think about the blood pressure and heart rate as you turn to the remainder of
your CV exam, using any clues they provide to refine your exam further. For
instance, is the pulse pressure large? If so, you will seek in the rest of your exam
further evidence of atherosclerotic disease or aortic insufficiency, the two most
common causes of a large systolic-diastolic pressure difference.

B. Peripheral pulses. Examine the force and regularity of the radial pulse. In fact,
this is a good way to begin your physical exam; it is unthreatening and provides a
first physical contact with the patient.

Examine the strength and integrity of all of the peripheral pulses.

For patients who may have a *cardiac catheterization*, the integrity of the femoral
and lower extremity pulses is important; it is these that will be examined after
the catheterization to assure that no major damage to the femoral artery

---

When performing cardiac auscultation
with the open bell, it is occasionally
difficult to distinguish between a fourth
heart sound (S_4) with a single first
heart sound (S_1), and a true split of S_1.
Since the S_4 is of low frequency while S_1
is of high frequency, the different ener-
gies generated by these sounds can be
used to differentiate the two without interrupting auscultation to change to the
diaphragm. If firm pressure is exerted
upon the bell, stretching the underlying
skin and making it taut (in function,
the skin becomes a stethoscope diaphragm), the S_4 will tend to diminish in
intensity, while the split S_1 will remain
of equal intensity. In essence, the low
energy generated by the low frequency
S_4 becomes insufficient to vibrate the
now taut skin, while the higher energy
S_1 is heard undiminished. A true split
of S_1 (mitral and tricuspid closures) will
generally be of the same intensity

whether heard with the bell or the diaphragm because of identical high fre-
quencies.

*When performing auscultation of the
heart, use a minimum of two patient positions.* Initially, the patient should be
screened in the supine position
with auscultation by both the bell and
diaphragm. The patient should then be
turned to a left lateral decubitus position (right shoulder elevated 45–60 degrees) and re-auscultated. The close
proximity of the heart to the left lateral
chest wall may permit detection of soft
heart sounds such as the S_3, S_4, or an
opening snap, or at the least may inten-
sify what was faintly heard in the
supine position. A third position (sitting
or leaning forward) may be desirable
when searching for an aortic diastolic
murmur.

Arthur A. Sasahara, M.D.

catheterized during the procedure has occurred. In patients with claudication, the inspection of the lower extremity pulses is obviously important. You can get an early and often accurate impression of the degree of vascular disease and the integrity of the cardiac contractile function by paying careful attention to the peripheral pulses.

II. Inspection

A. **Jugular venous pulse.** The height of the JVP column, a correlate of central venous (and therefore right heart) pressures, is determined (see Fig. 3-1 for details).

The contour of the JVP is then examined. This part of the CV exam is the most difficult. It is enough at first to be aware that a and v waves are visible in the venous pulsation in the neck (see Fig. 3-2). Note that the a and c components of the JVP tracing, as shown in Fig. 3-2, are so closely timed as to be seen as one impulse, referred to as the *a wave*. Note also that the a and v waves may be correlated with the events of the cardiac cycle and thus provide a physical exam correlate of a right heart pressure tracing.

B. **Point of maximal impulse**

1. When you look for a visible apex beat, describe its location in relation to the clavicle, axilla, and intercostal spaces or male nipple. If the PMI is absent, note this.

2. When you look for any other impulses, note how they are related to the PMI itself. Establish if and when extra impulses occur during the cardiac cycle, something to which you can return after auscultation.

III. Palpation

A. **Carotid pulse contour**

1. **Examine the carotid pulse.** Be careful while palpating the neck of an older patient or one with known arteriosclerotic disease.

2. **Consider the character of the pulse.** Is it strong? Does it have two apparent beats (characteristic of a *bisferiens pulse*)? Is there a short, "purring" sensation associated with the pulse that might be a *thrill*? Is the upstroke of the pulse normal, or is it delayed? Is the volume of the carotid pulse normal, or is it low volume? Are the carotid pulses symmetric? Are carotid thrills present? Is the carotid upstroke abnormally brisk with a larger than normal volume?

B. **Precordium**

1. **Feel for the apical impulse** and locate it anatomically. Think about the quality of the pulse. Does it strike your palm quickly? Does it stay pressed against the palm for a fraction longer than you had expected (a "slightly sustained impulse")? Is it vigorous or weak compared to what you have come to identify as normal? Is it absent? Is there a paradoxic motion to the apical impulse?

2. **Describe any other impulses present.** Do you feel the purring of a thrill? If you think so, it is important to check again, especially after ausculting, and describe anatomically where you feel it. Is S_1 or S_2 palpable? Can you feel the click of any valves closing? When in the cardiac cycle? Is there a right ventricular lift (felt as a sustained rise of the sternum or the chest wall just to the left of the sternum)?

IV. Auscultation

Auscultation is initially frustrating for everybody. You have to learn to think as you listen, to ignore one phase of the cardiac cycle and concentrate on another, to listen to each cardiac sound while excluding all others.

Standardize your **exam posture.** Approach the patient from his or her right side, even if doing so entails moving the bed from a wall or having the patient turn around in bed.

If you listen for a long time, you will sometimes prompt a patient to ask, "Is there anything wrong with my heart?" **Reassure your patient** that you are doing a careful exam, which is why you have listened for so long.

A. Vascular sounds. Always check for carotid bruits and transmitted murmurs.

B. Heart Sounds

1. The first goal of auscultation of the heart is **distinguishing systole from diastole.** This aim may sound simplistic, but it is not simple. Here are a few hints to make the distinction easier.

   a. Begin ausculting with the stethoscope held on the apex with one hand while your other hand gently feels the carotid pulse: the first heart sound, corresponding to closure of the atrioventricular valves and onset of systole, just precedes the carotid pulsation. This often can help you to distinguish S_1 (and therefore systole).

   b. In the absence of valvular pathology, the **intensity** of S_1 is greater than that of S_2 at the apex of the heart, while the intensity of S_2 is greater than that of S_1 at the base. (Listen at the aortic and pulmonic areas for the two components of S_2 and at the mitral area or PMI for S_1; see Fig. 3-3.)

   c. Although more subtle, the **pitch** of S_1 is discernibly lower than that of S_2 in most patients. Remember, high-frequency sounds are best heard with the diaphragm of your stethoscope, while low-frequency sounds are better appreciated with the bell.

   d. Remember that the PMI correlates with systole. This means that S_1 just precedes the onset of the apical impulse, which you may both see and feel with your hand and your stethoscope.

2. **"Inching."** Once you are oriented to systole and diastole, you can begin a systematic exam. It is helpful to base this assessment on an initial, routine path of movement of the stethoscope from the aortic to the pulmonic area and down the left sternal border to the mitral area (see Fig. 3-3). Develop a specific sequence at each step in this path in which the components of the cardiac cycle are systematically sought. Thus, at each stop along the inching "path," listen selectively to the following.

   a. S_1

   b. S_2

   c. Systole

   d. Diastole

   e. Extracardiac sounds

   It is crucial to learn to listen selectively to each of these components. Concentrate on *each* item individually in the above list, starting with S_1, at *each* step of the way. Inching will be lengthy, even tedious at first, but it will soon become routine, and is the best way to "hear" heart sounds effectively.

3. **Summary**

   a. Check for carotid bruits and transmitted murmurs.

   b. Orient yourself to systole and diastole.

   c. Starting at the aortic area and inching along the pathway outlined in **2,** listen for S_1, S_2, systolic sounds, diastolic sounds, and extracardiac sounds *one at a time.* Be patient and methodical.

   d. Practice drawing what you hear.

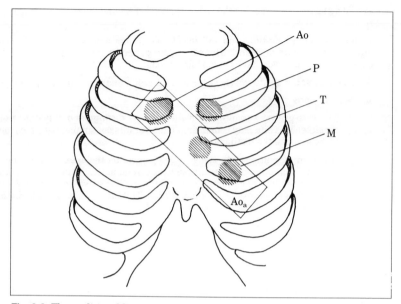

Fig. 3-3. The traditional listening areas for the aortic (Ao), pulmonic (P), tricuspid (T), and mitral (M) valves and associated murmurs. It is important to realize that cardiac murmurs, especially those associated with the aortic valve, are usually not confined to such discrete areas. An aortic murmur may radiate and be heard maximally in any portion of the "actual" aortic area (Ao$_a$), as shown above.

4. Third and fourth heart sounds

    a. The **third heart sound** is generated by the sudden termination of excessively rapid filling of the left ventricle, usually in the dilated heart. In mature patients, the S_3 is considered pathologic. Note that an S_3 may be heard in children and adolescents with normal hearts.

    The sound is a dull thud, lower in pitch than either an S_1 or S_2, heard in middiastole. It is timed after S_1 and S_2 roughly the way the third syllable ("eee") occurs in the word *Kentucky.*

    b. The **fourth heart sound** is generated by decreased ventricular compliance and the atrial systole, which ejects an atrial jet of blood against the stiff ventricle and thus generates a sound. An S_4 is occasionally heard in normal patients, but often implies myocardial disease.

    The sound is a low-pitched, short thud, higher in pitch than an S_3, but still somewhat less snapping in quality than a normal S_1 or S_2. It is timed preceding S_1 and S_2 roughly the way the first syllable ("ten") occurs in the word *Tennessee.*

C. Maneuvering and murmur analysis. Although a thorough description of murmur analysis is beyond the scope of this section, there are several basic points to remember at the start.

    1. Listen for murmurs with the patient first in the **supine position,** then the **left lateral decubitus position,** and then the **sitting position**. For example, the murmur of aortic insufficiency is often appreciated only with the patient sitting up and leaning slightly forward. Listen to a murmur at the apex with the patient in the left lateral decubitus position, which brings the heart closer to your stethoscope. This position can be very useful if you have trouble hearing any sounds, or if you suspect from the history that a diastolic rumble may be present (e.g., mitral stenosis).

    2. It is possible to alter the character of murmurs heard by **maneuvering** your patient in certain ways. *Maneuvering* is the physiologic alteration of venous return, peripheral arterial resistance, or cardiac output. For instance, the hand grip increases peripheral arterial resistance, which in turn decreases the gradient across the aortic valve in systole or increases the degree of mitral regurgitation. Therefore, an aortic systolic ejection murmur can sometimes be heard to decrease in intensity with the patient doing the hand grip maneuver, while that of mitral regurgitation may increase.

    Alterations in response to these maneuvers allow you to characterize the origin of the murmurs with greater accuracy. The basic maneuvers are either exertion-related or positional; examples of each type follow.

    a. Exertion-related maneuvers

        (1) Valsalva maneuver: decreases venous return.

        (2) Hand grip (isometric hand exercise): increases arterial pressure.

    b. Positional maneuvers

        (1) Sitting

        (2) Leg lifting: increases venous return.

        (3) Squatting: decreases venous return, increases arterial pressure.

    Always maneuver a patient who has a systolic murmur. Try to localize the murmur to the aortic or mitral valve in this manner, and attempt to explain the change in intensity of the murmur on the basis of the physiologic change resulting from your maneuver.

    Tables 3-2 to 3-5 provide a collection of points concerning auscultation of S_1, S_2, systolic murmurs, and diastolic murmurs. They are intended to be used as references in conjunction with your cardiac exam.

Table 3-2. Auscultation of heart sounds

Heart sound	Significance	Generated by	Best heard	Important auscultatory parameter(s)	Important pathophysiologic points
S_1	Normally present	Atrioventricular valve closure (mitral valve is major component)	At apex, with diaphragm or bell	**Intensity** of S_1 S_1 loud if it is better heard than S_2 in the aortic area	**Intensity** is determined by: 1. Position of the AV valves as systole begins. **Note:** This finding is correlated with the P-R interval. For example, a long P-R interval causes a softer S_1, since the AV valves have had longer to float to the closed position. 2. Rate of pressure rise in LV (dp/dt). 3. Morphologic changes in valve leaflet; these can diminish the intensity of S_1 by diminishing normal pliability. 4. Loud S_1 heard in mitral stenosis, the pressure gradient between left atrium and left ventricle keeping the mitral valve open until the onset of systole.
A_2	Normally present	Aortic valve closure	Throughout precordium, including pulmonic area (see Fig. 3-3)	**Intensity** of A_2 **Split** of A_2 from P_2 during inspiration	**Intensity** is determined by: 1. Morphologic status of valve. 2. Rate of end-systolic closure, which is related to

	Presence	Cause	Location	Features	Significance	Notes
P_2	Normally present	Pulmonic valve closure	Pulmonic area	**Intensity** of P_2 **Split** of P_2 from A_2 on inspiration		pressure present in aortic root and rate of pressure fall in LV ($-dp/dt$). **Split:** See P_2, below. **Intensity:** Same as A_2 (remember that P_2 is normally softer than A_2). **Split:** P_2 normally follows A_2 for two reasons (remember that split is not usually audible on expiration): 1. Prolonged ejection of RV due to increased compliance of pulmonary vasculature with inspiration i.e., *hangout* (the major reason for A_2-P_2 split). 2. Prolonged ejection of RV due to increased RV filling as inspiration augments venous return.
S_3	Pathologic; may be normal in children or young adults	Rapid filling and stretching of LV (LV often is abnormal)	At apex, with bell gently applied Soft, difficult to hear Follows S_1 and S_2 like the "y" follows "Kentuck" in "Kentucky"		**Presence** of S_3 a confirmation, rather than a fundamental sign, of heart disease	Present in conditions that may lead to rapid and increased ventricular filling, such as MR, AI, VSD, ASD, patent ductus arteriosus (PDA). Often an early sign of LV failure; a loud, prominent S_3, however, is associated with more severe failure.

Table 3-2 (Continued)

Heart sound	Significance	Generated by	Best heard	Important auscultatory parameter(s)	Important pathophysiologic points
S_4	Pathologic	Forceful atrial contraction into a stiffened LV (decreased LV compliance)	At apex, using bell, with patient in left lateral decubitus position Soft, difficult to hear Precedes S_1 and S_2 like the "a" precedes "penndix" in "appendix"	**Intensity** of S_4 important in evaluating hypertensive heart disease and failure	Present in conditions that may lead to reduced LV compliance, such as AS, hypertension, coronary artery disease, MI, hypertrophic cardiomyopathy. Sensitive indicator of hypertensive-associated heart failure; increased intensity and increased S_4-S_1 interval associated with more imminent failure.
Ejection clicks (aortic and pulmonic)	Pathologic change in valves or roots of great vessels	Stenosis of aortic or pulmonic valves, or dilatation of aorta or pulmonary artery	**Aortic:** apex, with diaphragm **Pulmonic:** left sternal border, second to third ICS, with diaphragm	**Presence** of an ejection click provides further clinical evidence for pathologic aortic or pulmonic valve	Closely follows S_1. Present in semilunar valve stenosis, hypertension, dilatation of either great vessel. **Pulmonic clicks** vary with respiration (best heard on expiration, may disappear with inspiration). In diagnosis of AS or PS, localizes pathologic change to valvular level.
Mid-to-late systolic clicks	Pathologic; often associated with mitral valve prolapse	Tensing of mitral chordae tendineae and/or snapping of the prolapsing leaflet	Apex, with diaphragm; may be heard at left sternal border as well	**Presence** of one or more mid-to-late systolic clicks most often associated with mitral valve prolapse	Often associated with a mid-to-late crescendo systolic murmur.

Table 3-3. Clinical points for S_1 and S_2

Heart sound	Auscultatory parameter	Clinical points
S_1	Split	**Split of S_1:** Of no clinical significance, but consider that you may be hearing an ejection click or S_4.
	Intensity	**Increased intensity:** Short P-R interval; mitral stenosis with valve still pliable. **Decreased intensity:** Long P-R interval; poor transmission, as in obesity and emphysema; mitral regurgitation; mitral stenosis with calcified, rigid valve. **Variable intensity:** Complete heart block; atrial fibrillation.

A_2/P_2	Split	**Wide or "fixed" split:** Failure of A_2-P_2 interval to close at end-expiration; may be a normal variant, in which case A_2-P_2 interval is easily heard to move with respiration, or may be due to two general causes:
		A. Early A_2 due to rapid emptying of the LV, as in VSD or MR.
		B. Late P_2 due to:
		  1. Right bundle branch block: ECG Dx to confirm.
		  2. Atrial septal defect: A true "fixed" splitting of S_2; may move slightly with expiration but will remain widely split.
		  3. Pulmonic stenosis: Secondary to prolonged RV ejection time.
		  4. Acute right heart overload: Sudden occurrence of an abnormally wide split, as in pulmonary embolism.
		Paradoxic split: Due to delayed closure of aortic valve; signifies pathology but is a difficult finding to hear. Two most common causes are (1) left bundle branch block (LBBB), confirmed by ECG and (2) aortic stenosis, indicative of a high degree of stenosis.
		Note: Paradoxic split is present in approximately 25% of patients with LBBB or AS. It is a specific but not a sensitive sign for these conditions.

	Intensity	**Accentuated A_2:** Systemic hypertension; aortic dilatation. **Diminished A_2:** Valvular AS; if AS is clinically present and A_2 is normal or increased, consider subvalvular outflow obstruction. **Accentuated P_2:** Pulmonary hypertension; may be normal in thin chested children or young adults. **Diminished P_2:** Pulmonic stenosis.

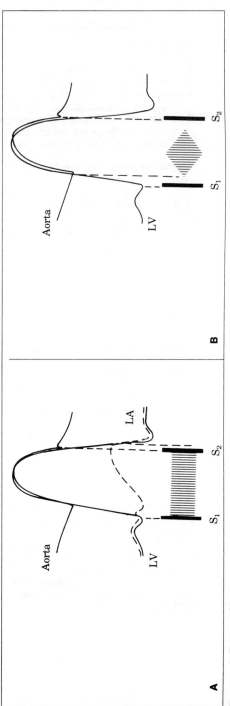

Fig. 3-4. A. Pansystolic murmur. B. Midsystolic ejection murmur.

Table 3-4. Systolic murmurs in adults

Systolic murmurs	Best appreciated	Associated signs	ECG	Chest x-ray	Clinical points
A. Systolic ejection murmur					
1. "Innocent" (be-nign)	Second to third left ICS	Normal, thin chest; pectus excavatum	Normal	Normal; pectus ex-cavatum; straight dorsal spine	Usually short, soft murmur. May vary with respi-ration. Usually not widely transmitted.

	Location	Physical findings	ECG	X-ray/Echo	Comments
					Must R/O valvular stenosis, high-output states, ASD, or signs of cardiomegaly to be confident of Dx of "innocent" murmur.
2. Physiologic	Second to third left ICS	Signs of anemia, pregnancy, fever, thyrotoxicosis	Normal	Normal	Often caused by high-output states.
3. Aortic stenosis, calcific	Aortic area with wide radiation. May be heard best at apex in older person	Diminished or absent A_2, S_4, LV heave. Carotid pulsus parvus and tardus, systolic thrill	LV hypertrophy (LVH)	↑ LV dimension, dilated ascending aorta, calcifications in valve	In older patients. Often diagnosed by delayed carotid pulse. Late peaking of murmur in systole correlates with more severe stenosis. Radiates to neck usually.
4. Aortic stenosis, congenital	Same as above	Usually normal A_2, ejection click, S_4, LV heave. Carotid pulsus parvus and tardus, systolic thrill	Same as above	↑ LV dimension, dilated ascending aorta	Noted in childhood or early adulthood. Presence of ejection click implies mobile, flexible valve.
5. Pulmonic stenosis	Second to third left ICS	Inspiratory EC, ↓ P_2, persistent split, thrill, left parasternal lift	RV hypertrophy (RVH), RA deviation (RAD)	Poststenotic dilatation of PA; prominent RV outflow track; normal peripheral lung vasculature	Intensity and duration of murmur correlate with severity of stenosis. Sometimes associated with other congenital cardiac malformations (e.g., ASD, VSD)

Table 3-4 (Continued)

Systolic murmurs	Best appreciated	Associated signs	ECG	Chest x-ray	Clinical points
6. Hypertrophic cardiomyopathy (IHSS)	Lower left sternal border (LLSB), apex	S_4, "spike and dome" bifid carotid pulse, LV heave. Murmur increases with Valsalva maneuver and upright posture	LVH, ST and T wave abnormalities. Abnormal Q waves (especially in inferolateral leads)	Normal, LVH LA enlargement if MR present.	May sound like AS at left sternal border (LSB), but be confused with murmur of MR when listening to apex. Maneuvering crucial to diagnosis. Echocardiographic confirmation with septal hypertrophy and systolic anterior motion of mitral valve (MV).
7. Atrial septal defect (ASD)	Pulmonic area	Wide, fixed split of S_2 Left parasternal lift or heave Associated with mid-diastolic rumble at LLSB if shunt is large (tricuspid flow murmur). Midsystolic pulmonary ejection murmur	Left axis deviation suggests a prinum ASD. Incomplete or complete right bundle branch block (RBBB), RVH, and right axis deviation (secundum defect). A leftward P wave axis suggests a sinus venosus ASD	Prominent pulmonary vasculature ↑ RV dimension	Systolic murmur of ASD due to RV and PA flow. Echocardiogram shows RV overload with paradoxic septal motion.

B. Pansystolic

1. Ventricular septal defect (VSD)	LLSB, high-pitched, harsh	Thrill, flow murmurs	Normal	Normal, small heart	Does not radiate to axilla. Begins with S_1. Small VSD may be best heard in second-third left ICS.
2. Mitral regurgitation, chronic	Apex, with axillary radiation; high-pitched, blowing	↓ S_1; S_3 often, LV heave. Vigorous, unsustained apical impulse	Left atrial abnormality. Atrial fibrillation common	↑ LA dimension. ↑ LV dimension. Calcified MV	Intensity of murmur *not* correlated with severity. Murmur continues to or through A_2. May be associated with early diastolic flow murmur.
3. Mitral regurgitation, acute	Apex, with axillary radiation	Same as above S_4	Normal	Normal heart size (unless long-standing changes). Pulmonary congestion	Acute MR may be a crescendo-decrescendo murmur that ends before A_2. Rupture of chordae tendineae or papillary muscle dysfunction is most commonly secondary to ischemic disease/MI.
4. Tricuspid regurgitation (TR)	LLSB, sternum, ± axillary radiation	Large systolic ("s" or "cV") waves in JVP. Pulsatile liver initially. Intensity increases with inspiration (Rivero-Carvello's sign). RV heave	Incomplete RBBB. Atrial fibrillation	↑ RA dimension. ↑ Vena cavae. Heart size increased	Murmur may continue through A_2 and P_2. Most common cause is functional dilatation accompanying RV failure

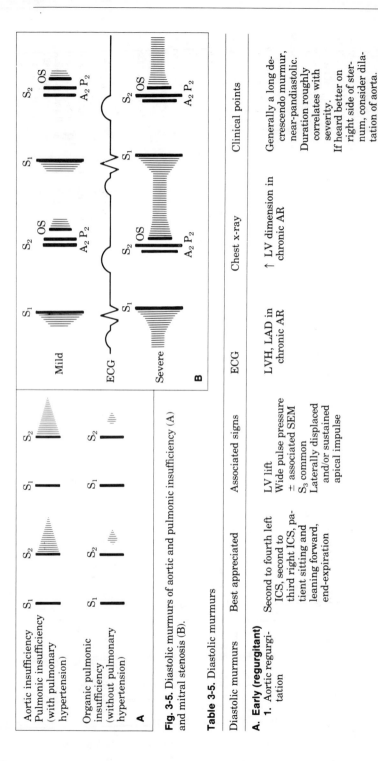

Fig. 3-5. Diastolic murmurs of aortic and pulmonic insufficiency (A) and mitral stenosis (B).

Table 3-5. Diastolic murmurs

Diastolic murmurs	Best appreciated	Associated signs	ECG	Chest x-ray	Clinical points
A. Early (regurgitant)					
1. Aortic regurgitation	Second to fourth left ICS, second to third right ICS, patient sitting and leaning forward, end-expiration	LV lift Wide pulse pressure ± associated SEM S₃ common Laterally displaced and/or sustained apical impulse	LVH, LAD in chronic AR	↑ LV dimension in chronic AR	Generally a long decrescendo murmur, near-pandiastolic. Duration roughly correlates with severity. If heard better on right side of sternum, consider dilatation of aorta. Apical diastolic rumble may accompany AR (Austin-Flint murmur)

2. Pulmonic regurgitation	Pulmonic area (third or fourth left ICS). Brief, diamond-shaped murmur if pulmonary pressures normal. If ↑ pulmonary pressures, more like AR.	RV lift Peripheral signs of AR absent Signs of LVH absent Signs of pulmonary hypertension may be present	RAD, RVH if pulmonary hypertension present. If not, rSr′ configuration in right precordial leads.	Avascular lung fields if pulmonary hypertension present	Usually secondary to pulmonary hypertension. Difficult to distinguish from AR: ↑ PA pressure and absence of peripheral signs of AR most helpful.

B. Mid-late Ventricular Filling*

1. Mitral stenosis	Apex, with bell Rumbling, low-pitched May be confined to small (half dollar–sized) area around PMI	"Snapping," ↑ S_1 Presystolic accentuation of murmur if no atrial fibrillation Opening snap RV heave and/or ↑ P_2 if associated pulmonary hypertension	RAD Broad, notched P waves (*P mitrale*)	↑ LA dimension (double density, right heart border) Kerley B lines	Left lateral decubitus may be helpful. Echocardiogram excellent for diagnosis.
2. Mitral regurgitation	Apex	↓ S_1 Associated systolic murmur of MR Usually S_3 LV lift	LAD, LVH	↑ LA dimension ↑ LV dimension	Diastolic **flow** murmur. May simulate murmur of MS but other signs of MS absent.
3. Left-to-right shunt (e.g., ASD, VSD; see above).	Apex	S_1 normal S_2-fixed split with ASD Systolic murmur of primary lesion associated (see Table 3-3)	Right bundle branch block (RBBB) with ASD Normal with VSD	↑ vascularity of lung fields	Due to increased pulmonary blood flow and therefore increased flow across MV (VSD, PDA) or increased flow across TV (ASD).

*Mid-late ventricular filling results from either blood rushing past rigid, fixed valves (as in MS) or increased flow past normal valves (as in MR).

The Clinical Laboratory

After you have taken the history and done the physical examination, you should, in most cases, be able to start answering the following questions:

1. What general types of disease processes am I being confronted with? What organ systems seem to be involved? Are the problems acute or chronic?
2. Based on the information that I have now, what are the top diagnoses on my differential diagnosis list?
3. How can I decide among these diagnoses?

Laboratory data are the final component in the initial data base that you will use to resolve questions of diagnosis and management. Note that, in general, there are two separate reasons for ordering a lab test: (1) to establish or exclude a **diagnosis**, or (2) to follow the **course** of a disease process. If you clarify in your own mind the specific goals of your lab analysis, you will cut down significantly on unnecessary pain, aggravation, and cost both to the patient and to yourself. You must always ask yourself how the results of a particular test will affect your clinical management decisions. The decision of whether or not to order a lab test is not always straightforward, especially if the purpose of the test is to rule out a disease that is already unlikely, or to give additional credence to a diagnosis that is already virtually certain. As a student, you will tend to err on the side of too much information, but you should still make an effort to justify each test that you order.

Time can be a physician's ally and a legitimate diagnostic test. The desire to reach a rapid diagnosis is often medically and economically justifiable. But in many instances, when the answer is not readily revealed, the pressure to find the diagnosis need not force the clinician to obtain more and more tests and to engage in ever more invasive procedures. Time allows a disease process to "declare itself" (or go away). The physician working in close communication with the patient can use time with little risk.

Thomas P. Stossel, M.D.

There is a magnificent quotation by Louis Pasteur, "In the Fields of Observation Chance Favors the Prepared Mind." One of the saddest features of academic medicine today is that we have adopted the intellectually narrow view that the only legitimate research activity is at the laboratory bench with beautifully designed narrow experiments in which the element of chance is eliminated to the greatest extent possible. The clinical scientist deliberately exposes himself to chance knowing that a random sampling of the uncountable experiments of nature will repeatedly present to his prepared mind unexpected phenomena that suddenly cast a bright light on previously unknown, but basic aspects of science. Perhaps the greatest clinical observer was Darwin, who, setting out on the *Beagle* on a voyage whose trajectory was not under his control and which was often altered by chance occurrences, could only be exposed to random and unexpected observations such as coral reefs and finches with different beaks on different islands. Yet, out of this random collection of astute clinical observations grew the theory of evolution.

Norman Geschwind, M.D.

Chaps. 4–9 cover the basics of the analysis and interpretation of six of the most important types of lab tests that you will encounter on the wards:

1. Hematologic Tests
2. Urinalysis
3. Common Serum Chemistries
4. Electrocardiography
5. Chest Radiology
6. Arterial Blood Gas Determination

Part A of each chapter outlines the indications for ordering the tests, the actual parts of each test battery, and the basis of the interpretation of the test results. Part B of each chapter contains useful principles and clinical tips concerning the performance and interpretation of the lab tests. Suggestions concerning the appropriate way to **record** the lab data are presented in Chap. 10, The Medical Write-Up and Progress Notes.

It must be emphasized that these chapters are only overviews. Their purpose is to provide a student orientation that emphasizes the essentials of clinical lab data collection and interpretation. Rather than presenting the entire differential diagnosis for lab findings, we have listed those with which the student should first be familiar. More in-depth presentations can be found in the texts listed in the References.

Sensitivity and Specificity

You must understand two test parameters in order to make best use of the clinical laboratory: **sensitivity** and **specificity**. Basically, *sensitivity* is the percent of time that, when a test indicates a disease's absence, the disease will in fact not be present (e.g., a sensitivity of 98% means that there will be only 2 false negatives for every 100 tested patients who actually have the disease). The mathematical expression for sensitivity is

$$\text{Sensitivity} = \frac{\text{true positive}}{\text{true positive} + \text{false negative}}$$

Specificity is the percent of time that a positive test result will correctly indicate that the patient does have the disease in question (thus a specificity of 95% means that there will be 5 false positives per 100 patients tested). The mathematical expression for specificity is

$$\text{Specificity} = \frac{\text{true negative}}{\text{true negative} + \text{false positive}}$$

It is important to realize the difference between these two test parameters: the presence of some degree of cardiac enlargement on the chest x-ray is a fairly sensitive test for congestive heart failure (i.e., most patients with CHF will show cardiac enlargement on their x-ray), but it is not a very specific test (because many other diseases also show this finding).

An interrelated concept that you should also keep in mind is **prevalence.** *Disease prevalence* in a screened population is defined as the total number of cases of a disease at a certain time in the designated population. Prevalence should be distinguished from *incidence*, the number of new cases of a specific disease during a specific period.

To understand how these concepts fit together, consider a hypothetic antenatal screening test designed to diagnose in utero a disease with a prevalence of 1 case per 1,000 births. If the test had a sensitivity of 100% and a specificity of 95%, testing of a population of 10,000 pregnant women might be expected to show 500 false positives and only 10 true positives. *The consequences are obvious: any clinical test is useful only to the extent of its specificity and sensitivity; these two parameters must be borne in mind in each instance of clinical decision-making.*

4

Hematologic Tests

Outline of Hematologic Tests

I. Reasons for ordering general hematologic tests. A **basic hematologic screen** (often referred to as a *complete blood count with differential white count*, or *CBC with diff*) is usually done on each patient admitted to the hospital. A set of **coagulation indices** is added whenever surgery is being considered or whenever there is a history of bleeding disorders. These tests provide useful information on four general categories of disease processes:

A. Hematopoietic problems, especially anemia and leukemia, both of which involve an alteration in the number and function of the blood cells.

B. Systemic diseases, especially renal and liver disease, which alter the hematologic environment, causing morphologic and functional changes in the blood cells.

In looking at a *peripheral blood smear*, I often spend as much time finding the appropriate field as actually examining the cells since one can miss clear-cut abnormalities or observe artifactual abnormalities when viewing a bad area. I first look at the blood smear with the naked eye and determine where it is thin and smooth. This should be toward the center of a coverslip smear and toward the feathered edge of a push-type smear made on a microscopic slide. The appropriate area is where the red blood cells are close to one another but are rarely touching and where most of the red cells have soft hypochromic centers; when two cells touch each other they usually appear to be spherocytes, but this is an artefact of the preparation.

Stephen H. Robinson, M.D.

Although most automatic cell counters will give values for the MCV and MCH, it is important to examine the peripheral blood smear for size and color intensity. The values given by the lab are means and will miss individuals with two populations of red cells. The best way to assess the size of the red cell is to relate it to the nucleus of a small lymphocyte; they should be the same. The normochromic red cell has a pale center that is one-third the diameter of the cell.

Harvey J. Cohen, M.D.

Definitive lab tests to diagnose *iron deficiency anemia* (Fe/TIBC tests) are expensive and inaccurate and take time to perform. A simple screening method involves holding a spun "crit" tube up against a white background. Normal individuals have an amber colored serum, while those with iron deficiency have a clear serum. Hyperbilirubinemia can obscure this test, but not much else can confuse you.

Jeffrey M. Lipton, M.D.

Table 4-1. CBC: Normal values and range

Hct: Men: 47 ± 7.0
Women: 42 ± 5.0
Hgb: Men: 14–18 gm/100 ml
Women: 12 –16 gm/100 ml
MCV: 85–100 μm³; **MCH:** 28–31 μμg; **MCHC:** 30–35%
RBC: Diameter: 7.3–7.5 μ
Men: 4.2–5.4 × 10⁶ cells/mm³
Women: 3.6–5.0 × 10⁶ cells/mm³
Reticulocytes: 0.5–1.5%
WBC: Total: 4–11 × 10³ cells/mm³
Diff
PMN: 40–75%
Lymphocytes: 15–45%
Eosinophils: 1–6%
Basophils: 0–2%
Monocytes: 1–10%
Platelets: 145–375 × 10³/mm³
PT: Depends on lab; usually ~ 12–14 sec. Always given with control; should be within 2 secs of control.
PTT: Depends on lab; usually 25–45 sec. Always given with control; should be within 4 secs of control.
ESR: Wintrobe
Men: 0–5 mm/hr
Women: 0–15 mm/hr
Westergren
Men: 0–15 mm/hr
Women: 0–20 mm/hr

C. **Infection,** which often results in increased total leukocyte count. Depending on whether this increase is predominantly toward early myeloid forms ("shift to the left") or toward lymphoid forms, one can draw a general conclusion about the nature of the insult.

D. **Hemostatic problems,** which often manifest themselves through a protracted clotting time on one or more of the clotting screens.

II. **Parts of a routine hematologic screening battery**

A. **Complete blood count and indices.** In most hospitals, the CBC is a mechanized spectrophotometric analysis of an anticoagulated specimen of the peripheral blood. It results in a reasonably accurate estimate of the number, size, and hemoglobin content of the erythrocytes. The reported results include the hematocrit (Hct), the red blood cell count (RBC) and white blood cell count (WBC), the hemoglobin concentration (Hgb), and the red cell morphologic indices (mean corpuscular volume [MCV], mean corpuscular hemoglobin [MCH], mean corpuscular hemoglobin concentration [MCHC]). See Table 4-1 for normal values.

B. **Differential white cell count.** The diff, usually done by a technician, is a quantitation of the proportions of different types of leukocytes seen on a sample of several hundred cells during inspection of the smear of the patient's peripheral blood. It is reported as the percent of total leukocytes made up by each individual type of white cell.

C. **Blood smear analysis.** The smear analysis, usually done on an informal basis by the technician performing the diff, involves an inspection under high magnification of the size and appearance of the red and white cells. It is often reported as a "comment" on the hematology results lab slip.

D. **Platelet count and clotting indices.** The platelet count and the clotting indices are mechanized tests that screen for hemostatic problems. The usual battery of hemostatic tests includes, in addition to a platelet count, a prothrombin time (PT) and a partial thromboplastin time (PTT). Other clotting factor tests may be ordered if the results of the initial screening battery are abnormal, or if a specific defect is suspected.

E. **Erythroid sedimentation rate.** The erythroid sedimentation rate (ESR) is a nonspecific test that is loosely correlated with the serum levels of fibrinogen and globulin. Although not really part of a general hematologic screen, the ESR is often ordered and reported as part of the hematologic work-up. It is especially useful in screening for malignancy, connective tissue disorders, and infection, and in following the course of chronic inflammatory disease states.

III. **Analyzing and interpreting results of hematologic tests**

A. **Complete blood count and indices**

1. The **hematocrit** and the **red blood cell count** are reflections of the concentration of erythrocytes in the blood. Although the hematocrit will usually indicate whether or not the patient has some degree of anemia, you must analyze it together with the hemoglobin concentration and the red cell indices in order to determine the class of anemia (e.g., hypochromic microcytic vs. normochromic normocytic) and thereby gain insight into the etiology of the anemia.

2. The **red cell indices** represent average values for the size and hemoglobin content of the red cells. They are calculated as follows:

$$\text{MCV} = \frac{\text{Hct (\%)} \times 10}{\text{RBC (millions/mm}^3)}$$

(normal range 85–100 μm^3)

$$\text{MCH} = \frac{\text{Hgb (gm/100 ml)} \times 10}{\text{RBC (millions/mm}^3)}$$

(normal range 28–31 $\mu\mu g$)

$$\text{MCHC} = \frac{\text{Hgb (gm/100 ml)}}{\text{Hct (\%)}}$$

(normal range 30–35%)

Fig. 4-1 represents an approach to the differential diagnosis of anemia based on the red cell indices and the reticulocyte count.

3. The **total white blood cell count** is useful both as a diagnostic tool and in following the course of diseases. Shown below are the most common types of processes associated with increased and decreased WBC values.

a. Processes consistent with **WBC decrease**

(1) Infections, especially overwhelming bacterial infection, septicemia, and so on.

(2) Viral infections: infectious mono, hepatitis, influenza.

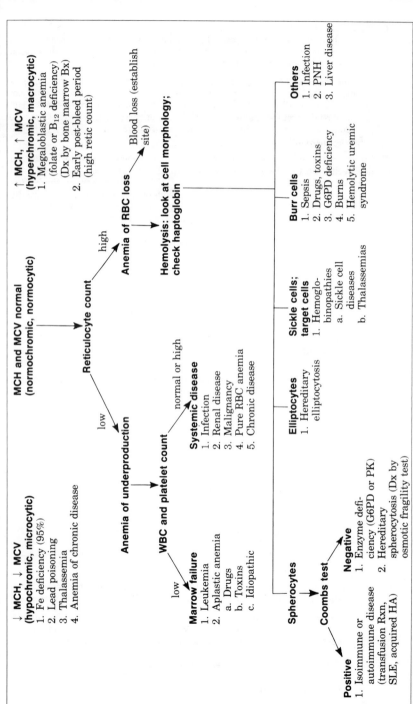

Fig. 4-1. Approach to the diagnosis of anemia on the basis of red cell indices.

(3) Drugs, e.g., sulfonamides, antibiotics.

(4) Radiation and cytotoxic chemotherapy.

(5) Hematologic diseases: pernicious and aplastic anemia.

b. Processes consistent with **WBC increase**

(1) Acute infections: pneumonia, meningitis, rheumatic fever, septicemia.

(2) Intoxications: uremia, acidosis, eclampsia, chemical poison, drugs (e.g., prednisone).

(3) Hemorrhage, RBC hemolysis, myeloproliferative diseases.

(4) Leukemia.

B. Differential white blood cell count. The diff reflects the response of the bone marrow hematopoietic feedback systems to physiologic and pathologic processes. Although the diff is usually too nonspecific to suggest an exact diagnosis, it is a fairly convenient way of following the course of many types of diseases, especially infections and neoplastic processes. For these two types of disease, it is also useful to analyze the maturity of the various leukocyte types. In general, high numbers of immature cells in the peripheral blood reflect either a "push on the marrow" to produce these cells in large quantities (e.g., a common manifestation of a bacterial pneumonia is a "shift to the left" with high numbers of immature granulocytes [bands] seen on the diff) or a developmental arrest suggesting primary hematologic disease. Shown below are the disease processes associated with increases and decreases in the proportions of the various specific leukocyte types reported on the diff. **An erythrocyte is shown next to cells 2–5 for size comparison.**

1. Granulocytes
(polymorphonuclear [PMNs])
Increase consistent with infections (endocarditis, pneumonia, septicemia), granulocytic leukemia, burns, eclampsia, RBC destruction.
Decrease consistent with drugs, viral infections, bone marrow invasion or aplasia.

2. Lymphocytes
Increase consistent with infections (mononucleosis, infectious hepatitis, and other viral infections), TB, lymphocytic leukemias.

3. Monocytes
Increase consistent with monocytic leukemia, TB, myeloproliferative disorders, HD, lipid storage diseases, SBE, collagen disease (RA, SLE), chronic infection or inflammation.

4. Eosinophils
Increase consistent with allergic disorders (asthma, hay fever), parasitic infection, collagen vascular disease, pernicious anemia, Addison's disease.
Decrease consistent with hypercortisolism, infections.

5. Basophils
Increase consistent with CML, polycythemia, myeloid metaplasia.

C. Blood smear analysis. While the diff is concerned primarily with the association between disease processes and the **proportions** of various leukocytes seen in the blood, the blood smear analysis is concerned primarily with the association between disease processes and red and white blood cell **morphology.** Since the morphology of blood cells is a function of both **intracellular events** and **extracellular environment,** analysis of the peripheral smear is a simple and powerful screening test for assessing systemic disease as well as cellular metabolic pathology.

Shown below are the most significant abnormalities commonly noted in red cells and leukocytes (together with the pathophysiologic basis for these abnormalities) and the common differential diagnoses associated with them.

Abnormality	Significance	Seen in
1. Red cell abnormal forms		
A. Target cells	Increase in surface-volume ratio	Liver disease, hemoglobinopathies, thalassemia, Fe^{2+} deficiency anemia, post-splenectomy states
B. Spherocytes	Decrease in surface-volume ratio	Hereditary spherocytosis, autoimmune hemolytic anemia
C. Siderocytes (need Fe^{2+} stain)	Cells with deposits of iron-containing granules	Postsplenectomy states, severe hemolysis, sideroblastic anemia
D. Basophilic stippling	Aggregations of defective ribosomes	Lead poisoning
E. Howell-Jolly bodies	Nuclear fragments	Postsplenectomy states, megaloblastic anemia
F. Macroovalocyte	Defective RBC maturation	Megaloblastic anemia, bone marrow failure
G. Polychromatophilic and immature erythroid forms in peripheral blood	Immature red cells	Any stress erythropoiesis (e.g., hemolysis, chronic hemorrhage)
H. Sickled cells	Molecular defect in hemoglobin beta-chain	Sickle cell anemias (SS, SC, S-thal)
I. Helmet cells	Sheared and traumatized erythrocytes	Microangiopathic hemolytic anemias (e.g., DIC), malignant hypertension, uremia, burns
J. Teardrop cells	Deformed RBC membrane	Marrow infiltration, myeloproliferative syndromes, extramedullary hematopoiesis
K. Reticulocytes (need special stain)	RNA network visible in very young RBC	Any state of high erythropoietic activity, e.g., post-bleed, post-Fe^{2+} treatment for anemia

Abnormality	Significance	Seen in
2. White cell abnormal forms		
A. Toxic granules in PMN	Reaction to sepsis	Infection or inflammatory disease
B. Dohle bodies in PMN	Ribosome-containing immature granules	Infection, burns
C. Hypersegmented PMN	Abnormality of nuclear division or chromatin	Folate or B_{12} deficiency, marrow failure
D. Auer rods (in myeloblasts)	Clumped granule material	AML, AMMoL
E. Atypical lymphocytes (vacuolated cytoplasm; lobulated monocytoid nucleus; nucleoli)	Activated T cells or lymphoblasts	Infectious mononucleosis, viral infections, immunologic reactions
F. Immature granulocytes in peripheral blood	Immature granulocytes	Infections, leukemoid reaction, leukoerythroblastic reactions, AML, CML
G. Bacteria in PMN	Phagocytosed bacteria	Severe infection

D. Platelet count and clotting indices. The platelet count and clotting indices are reflections of the state of the patient's hemostatic systems. Although the routine hemostasis screen includes the platelet count, the PT, and the PTT, it is obvious that these tests are quite different: the platelet count represents the amount of a hemostasis constituent (remember that platelet function is measured by a bleeding time), while the PT and PTT assess clotting factor activity (the amounts of specific factors are measured radioimmunologically). Thus, while normal platelet count and clotting indices suggest that the patient has normal hemostasis, an abnormal test result usually requires a more rigorous work-up to define the exact abnormality.

Shown below are common disease states associated with high or low platelet counts. Fig. 4-2 reviews the coagulation cascade and illustrates which factors are measured by the PT and PTT, while Table 4-2 summarizes the diagnosis of specific factor deficiencies, disorders that may lead to abnormal PT or PTT values.

Abnormal platelet counts   **Increased with** malignancy, myeloproliferative diseases, postsurgery or postsplenectomy states, collagen disorders (RA), Fe^{2+} deficiency anemia, bleeding, acute infection, primary thrombocytosis.

Note: platelet is acute phase reactant.

Decreased with ITP, marrow invasion or aplasia, hypersplenism.

Abnormal function aspirin therapy.

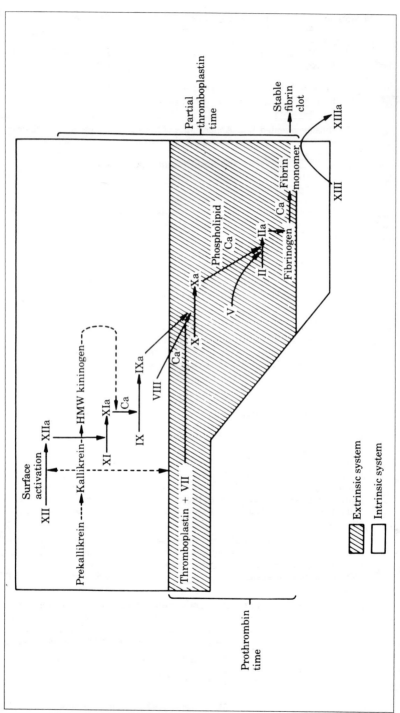

Fig. 4-2. Clotting sequence. (Reprinted with permission from H. H. Friedman, *Problem-Oriented Medical Diagnosis* [3rd ed.]. Boston: Little, Brown, 1983.)

Table 4-2. Diagnosis of clotting factor deficiencies

	Deficient factor	PT	PTT	Platelet count	Bleeding time
I	Fibrinogen	A	A	N	N
II	Prothrombin	A	A	N	N or A
III	Tissue thromboplastin	—	—	—	—
IV	Calcium	—	—	—	—
V	Labile factor	A	A	N	N or A
VI	(Not assigned)	—	—	—	—
VII	Stable factor	A	N	N	N
VIII	Antihemophilic globulin	N	A	N	N
IX	Christmas factor	N	A	N	N
X	Stuart-Prower factor	A	A	N	N or A
XI	Plasma thromboplastin antecedent	N	A	N	N
XII	Hageman factor	N	A	N	N
XIII	Fibrin stabilizing factor	N	N	N	N
	Fletcher factor	N	A	N	N
	Fitzgerald factor	N	A	N	N
	Von Willebrand's disease	N	N or A	N	N or A
	Thrombocytopenia	N	N	A	N or A
	Functional platelet defect	N	N	N or A	A
	Vascular defect	N	N	N	N or A

N = normal; A = abnormal.
Source: From H. H. Friedman, *Problem-Oriented Medical Diagnosis* (2nd ed.). Boston: Little, Brown, 1979. Reprinted with permission.

E. Erythroid sedimentation rate. Because it is so nonspecific, the ESR is most useful in deciding among sets of disease states that may have similar presentations but different degrees of inflammatory reaction and antibody formation. For instance, the ESR may be useful in deciding between rheumatoid arthritis (increased) and degenerative joint disease (normal).

Shown below are the common diseases associated with increased or decreased ESR values.

Abnormal ESR values   **Increased with** acute MI, infection, rheumatic fever, malignancy, myeloma, collagen diseases (RA, SLE), pregnancy, tuberculosis, active hepatitis, inflammatory necrosis.

Decreased with sickle cell anemia, polycythemia, CHF, DIC, trichinosis.

B   **Practical Points Concerning**
                                         Hematologic Tests

I. Complete blood count and indices

A. Remember that the **red cell indices** are mechanically calculated as the average of a great many cells. Look at the smear to confirm that the erythrocytes are morphologically homogenous. Multiple erythrocyte populations with mathematically compensatory abnormalities may result in falsely normal results.

B. You can get a good estimate of the hematocrit by multiplying the hemoglobin × 3 (e.g., a Hgb of 10 predicts a Hct of 30). Also note that, because the MCHC depends on these interlinked Hgb and Hct values, it will almost always be ~ 33 (and is therefore relatively useless).

C. When discussing a patient's problems, always state the **type of anemia** (e.g., hypochromic microcytic). Strictly speaking, anemia is not a disease it is a family of diseases. You must specify the nature of the anemia.

D. Remember that the most common etiology of anemia is **iron deficiency**, which results in microcytic hypochromic erythrocytes. This is a very common finding, especially among menstruating women.

E. **Bleeding** can produce either a normochromic normocytic or hyperchromic macrocytic picture. In a patient with a normal hematocrit who becomes anemic over the course of a few hours, always think about an acute bleed.

F. In working up an anemia of unknown etiology, always guaiac the stool to rule out **GI bleeding.**

II. Differential white cell count

A. The diff is a relatively expensive test and is probably overordered in most hospitals. You can perform your own mini-diff simply by looking at the smear and quickly scanning the field for **PMN band forms.** If there are more than a few percent bands, the diff is probably left-shifted.

B. Remember to look at the **eosinophil count** in patients with allergic disorders. (A mnemonic for remembering which problems are associated with high eosinophil levels: **worms, wheezes, weird diseases.**)

III. Blood smear analysis

A. It is worth learning to do a **Wright stain** of the peripheral blood for some patients you work up. The best way to learn how to do this is to watch a technician or hematologist a few times. It is impossible to interpret a poorly made smear.

B. Learn to scan the **microscopic field** with an eye to four parameters: (1) cell size, (2) cell shape, (3) nuclear shape, and (4) cytoplasmic inclusions. As in all lab tests, you should think about the patient's clinical history while looking at the smear. (Is there a history of liver disease? If so, does the peripheral smear show acanthocytosis?) Ask yourself not only, "What do I see?," but also, "What do I not see?"

C. Make friends with the **technicians** in the hematology lab. They will usually be happy to look at a smear with you, and they usually have excellent eyes for detail.

IV. Platelet count and clotting indices

A. Specific factor deficiency tests are expensive and should not be ordered routinely. Remember that abnormalities on clotting screens are more commonly due to **systemic disease** (e.g., liver failure) than to congenital factor deficiencies.

B. Because the platelets are important in the **primary hemostatic reaction** but play virtually no role in clotting, a hemophiliac with normal platelet levels will usually have a normal bleeding time.

V. Erythroid sedimentation rate. Remember that there are two different ways to test the ESR (the Wintrobe and the Westergren methods) and that the normal values are different for men and women. Always check what the technicians in your hospital lab consider a normal ESR.

I. Indications for the urinalysis

   A. An **admission urinalysis** (U/A) will be done routinely on virtually every patient. This urine sample may have been collected and sent to the hospital lab before the patient arrives on the hospital floor. In this situation, it is not uncommon for the medical student or house officer to perform a second urinalysis as part of the initial patient work-up. Centrifuge, microscope, and stains are usually provided on the wards for this purpose.

   B. In **following a patient** who has disease of the urinary tract or certain metabolic diseases such as diabetes mellitus, a partial or complete urinalysis is often done daily or every other day. Because urinary tract infections are so common, serial urinalyses are also done on patients with sepsis or unexplained fevers.

II. Parts of the urinalysis. There are nine basic parts to a complete urinalysis:

   A. Specific gravity

   B. Appearance

   C. pH*

   D. Protein*

   E. Sugar*

   F. Ketones*

   G. Blood*

   H. Sediment analysis

   I. Gram stain for bacteria (see Colorplates A, B, and C)

Fig. 5-1 is a flow diagram of the entire urinalysis, which can be done in 10 to 15 minutes.

In instances where urinary tract infection is suspected, a bacterial **culture and sensitivity** screen is added to the above list.

*A test done by dipstick.

For the patient with renal disease, the evaluation of the *urinary sediment* is not a laboratory procedure but rather an integral part of the physical examination to be performed by the physician, like listening to the chest or palpating the abdomen. Only then can the physician appreciate the often inconspicuous admixtures of cells and casts that define parenchymal disease: *red cell casts* indicating proliferative glomerular disease, *hyaline casts* indicating proteinuria, *white cell casts* indicating interstitial disease, *broad casts* indicating tubular atrophy, *waxy casts* indicating nephron death.

Warren E. Grupe, M.D.

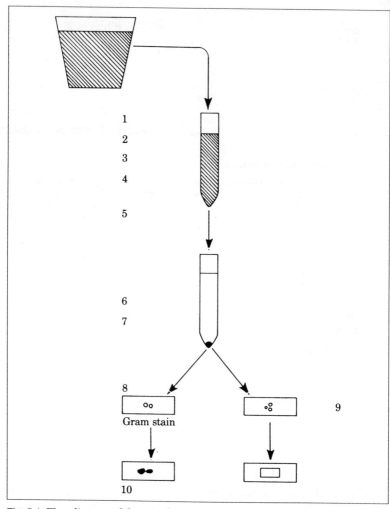

Fig. 5-1. Flow diagram of the urinalysis, which is performed as follows:

1. Pour 5–10 ml into a conical test tube.
2. Check specific gravity in remainder.
3. Using dipstick, check for pH, protein, sugar, ketones, and heme in remainder as well.
4. If UTI is suspected, check Gram stain of *unspun* specimen.
5. Spin at 1,000–2,000 rpm for 3–5 min.
6. Pour off supernatant.
7. Resuspend pellet in the 1–2 drops of urine that will remain after decanting by flicking bottom of test tube several times with your fingers or by knocking it against counter top.
8. Place 2 drops on a glass slide to dry for Gram stain.
9. While Gram stain preparation dries, place 2–3 drops of sediment on another glass slide; cover the second slide immediately with cover slip.
10. Examine sediment under high-dry power (never oil). Examine Gram stain slide under oil.

III. Interpreting the urinalysis

A. Specific gravity

1. **Normal range** 1.001–1.035, with urine isotonic to plasma (285–295 mOsm) 1.010–0.012. The specific gravity (SG) is used as in indirect measure of the kidney's ability to concentrate the urine. If a first morning specimen is SG 1.025 or greater, it is generally taken as evidence of adequate concentrating ability.

2. **False elevations** of SG may occur with iodinated contrast material, excessive glucose, and massive proteinuria.

B. Appearance. Urine is often described as "straw" or "yellow." Shown below are common causes of unusual color or turbidity:

Urine appearance	Possible cause
Red-brown	Hemoglobin, myoglobin, bile pigments, blood, food dyes
Yellow-red	Pyridium, vegetable or phenolphthalein cathartics
Blue or green	Beets, methylene blue in IV
Dark or black	Porphyrins, malanin
Turbid	Frequently secondary to urates or phosphates (benign), RBCs, WBCs
Foamy	Protein, bile acids

C. pH. The **normal range** of urine pH is **4.5–8.5.** In the appropriate clinical setting an alkaline urine may suggest either a urinary tract infection with a urea-splitting organism (e.g., *Proteus, Klebsiella, Escherichia coli*) or bicarbonate excretion (e.g., renal tubular acidosis). To differentiate these two possibilities, the alkaline urine is **boiled.** If a urea-splitting organism is present, NH_3 will vaporize and (1) pH paper held above the boiling urine will turn alkaline colors, (2) the pH of the specimen will fall after it is boiled, and (3) ammonia odor will be apparent.

D. Protein. The normal amount of urine protein is less than 50 mg/day. Persistent proteinuria is a highly significant finding. However, the dipstick will record false positives with strongly alkaline urine and, in uncertain cases, urine protein is better tested using a combination of heat and acetic acid.

1. **Heat and acetic acid**

   a. Simply add several drops of glacial acetic acid (or 3% acetic acid) to a test tube containing 2–4 ml of urine, so that the pH < 5; warm gently to dissolve any turbidity; and then boil the upper part of the tube over the Bunsen burner.

   b. Compare the turbidity of the urine in the upper half to that of the lower unboiled portion. This gives a rough idea of the degree of proteinuria.

2. Note that protein in urine may be either **normal** serum proteins (indicating glomerular permeability or renal tubular disorders) or **abnormal** serum proteins (suggesting possible plasma cell dyscrasia). In multiple myeloma, Bence-Jones (B-J) proteins will give a negative dipstick result about 50% of the time. Therefore, a positive heat–acetic acid test and negative dipstick may indicate B-J proteins and multiple myeloma.

E. Sugar. No detectable glucose (negative dipstick) is considered a normal result. This test is the main method for diagnosis of the common disease **diabetes mellitus.** The dipstick is extremely sensitive and specific for glucose, since the reaction relies on the enzyme glucose oxidase. However, the results are qualitative.

In situations where a quantitative assessment of urine glucose is desirable (as in monitoring how much glucose your patient with diabetes is spilling—an indirect way of assessing the efficacy of insulin therapy), use the Clinitest tablets and the dilution method explained with the bottle.

F. Ketones. The dipstick (and the Acetest tablets that are sometimes used) measure only acetoacetic acid and acetone (*not* beta-hydroxybutyrate).

Recall that ketosis is seen in cases of **extreme fasting** or **starvation** and **alcoholism** as well as **poorly controlled diabetes mellitus.**

G. Blood. Hematuria is virtually always significant. See Table 5-1 for a discussion of RBCs in urine.

H. Sediment.

1. **Preparation** (Fig. 5-1)

   a. Turn condenser down to distance it farther from slide. Use reduced light.

   b. Use low power first.

   c. Examine near the four edges of the cover slip where casts accumulate.

   d. Go to high power for cell counts and identification of casts and debris.

   e. If the urine specimen is purulent or bloody, remember to look at an unspun specimen first.

   f. You may want to stain the sediment to visualize better the various elements present. The most useful stain for this purpose is the Sternheimer-Malbin stain (crystal violet-Safarin 0); use 2 drops for each 0.5 ml sediment.

2. **Common errors** leading to unsatisfactory urine sediment examination

   a. Contamination of collecting vessel with foreign material.

   b. Inadequately resuspended sediment.

   c. Failure to use both high- and low-power magnification.

   d. Too much light.

   e. Dried specimen.

3. **Sediment analysis**

   a. Cells in the urine sediment

      (1) Cell counts. Count RBCs, WBCs, epithelial cells, and bacterial cells present in a typical high-power field (HPF).

      (2) Interpretation of cellular sediment. Table 5-1 lists the cell types found in the urine sediment and their significance.

   b. Casts in the urine sediment are often difficult to interpret. Remember that no casts are pathognomonic for a specific renal parenchymal change, and that they may be absent in any of a number of nephropathies.

      Casts are so called because they are casts of the nephron. They are distinguished from other debris by **smooth, parallel sides** (which may show the trapezoidal narrowing of the collecting system). Table 5-2 lists the various types of casts found in the urine and their clinical significance. These casts are illustrated in Fig. 5-2.

   c. Crystals in the urine sediment are due to precipitated chemicals and cellular debris. Some of the more common types of crystals are illustrated in Fig. 5-2. Their interpretation depends on the clinical presentation involved.

Table 5-1. Cell types in the urine sediment

Cell type	Normal range	Clinical points
RBC	0–3/HPF	**Cystitis** is the most frequent cause of hematuria, although slight hematuria often occurs secondary to exertion, trauma, or febrile illness. **Yeast cells** may be confused with RBCs. To distinguish between the two, RBCs may be lysed with 2–3 drops of acetic acid under cover slip (yeast cells will not lyse).
WBC	0–5/HPF	**Polymorphonuclear leukocytes** are the most common form of WBCs observed. If seen, and routine cultures × 2 are negative, send culture to be tested for tubercle bacilli.
Epithelial	0–2/HPF	**Epithelial cells** increase with tubular damage or heavy proteinuria.
Bacteria (see Colorplate D, 9)		Presence of bacteria on Gram stain of *un*spun specimen correlates well with culture growth of $\geq 10^5$ organisms (i.e., indicates presence of urinary tract infection). Send specimen for "culture and sensitivity" if suspicious. If culture comes back with between 10^4 and 10^5 organisms of a single type, reculture it; you must culture specimen at least twice to obtain >90% chance of documenting infection.

Table 5-2. Casts in urine sediment

Cast type	Clinical points
Hyaline (translucent albumin) cast	The majority of casts seen in normal urine are hyaline. Since their refractile index is close to that of water, they are difficult to see unless light is reduced. A few hyaline casts/HPF may be normal.
WBC cast	Use acetic acid to prove that these are not RBC casts (acetic acid will lyse RBCs). WBC casts indicate inflammation in kidney parenchyma (often pyelonephritis).
RBC cast	Must search entire perimeter of cover glass if you suspect RBC casts. They are most consistent with glomerular inflammation or ischemic injury.
Granular-waxy cast	Granular casts are so named because of their granular appearance under microscope. They are thought to be degenerating cellular casts, usually epithelial in origin. If they have a red tinge, R/O RBC casts.
Broad cast	Broad casts probably originate in wide collecting duct. They are formed when flow rate is low. They often have ominous prognostic significance.

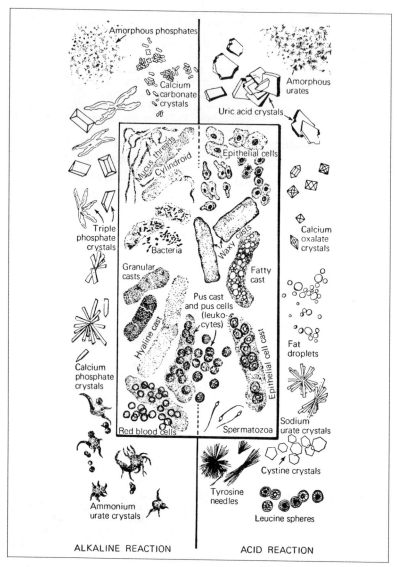

ALKALINE REACTION   ACID REACTION

Fig. 5-2. Microscopic examination of urine sediment. (Reprinted with permission from M. A. Krupp, et al., *Physician's Handbook* [19th ed.]. Los Altos, Calif.: Lange, 1979.)

B	**Practical Points Concerning the Urinalysis**

I. Ordering and performing the urinalysis

A. Since a urinalysis takes only about 10 minutes to perform, do a urinalysis every day on your patients with active **renal tract disease.** You will be able to follow the course of the disease more closely and present the case more forcefully in rounds if you can correlate the clinical history with the urinalysis findings.

B. Beware of assuming that urine samples indicate urinary tract disease if they are entirely normal except for **large numbers of red blood cells.** Menstruating women often contaminate their urine sample accidentally and Foley catheters commonly cause hematuria, while individuals seeking narcotics may deliberately mix blood into their urine to feign a kidney stone and receive pain medications. If you are suspicious about a urine sample, supervise its collection yourself.

C. Always Gram stain and culture the urine if your patient develops a **fever of unknown origin.** Surgical patients or any patients who have had urethral instrumentation often develop urinary tract infections.

II. Interpreting the urinalysis results

A. If you are having trouble identifying cells in the urine sediment, take a buccal scraping from your mouth and suspend it in a drop of the urine. Observing this sample should give you an idea of the size and appearance of epithelial cells at whatever magnification you are using.

B. In a patient with diabetes that is not well controlled, you will want to dipstick each urine sample and attempt to correlate the urine sugars with the blood sugars and other changes in the patient's clinical condition. It is extremely useful to discover a reasonable correlation between blood sugar and urine dipstick sugar.

6

Serum Chemistry Tests

A

Annotated Outline of Serum Chemistry Tests

I. **Indications for ordering serum chemistry tests.** Serum chemistry tests have become an important part of modern medical management. In general, they are ordered for four reasons:

    A. To aid in medical **diagnosis.**

    B. To allow the physician to **follow the course** of a problem or treatment regimen.

    C. To monitor **fluid and electrolyte balance.**

    D. To **screen for occult disease.**

Most patients will have a battery of 6–20 serum chemistry tests done as part of a standard admission profile. Serum chemistries tested will usually include, as a minimum, a set of electrolytes (Na, K, Cl, HCO_3), BUN, serum creatinine, and serum glucose. Other tests are added depending on hospital admission protocols and the nature of the patient's problem.

Listed below are 20 of the most important serum tests together with short lists of common diseases associated with abnormal values for these tests. Some essential points related to the interpretation of specific tests are included here. Further clinical points related to serum chemistries in general are included in part B of this chapter.

II. **Interpreting serum chemistry tests.** The following lists of physiologic and pathologic conditions associated with lab abnormalities include only some of the more common serum chemistry correlates. For a more complete treatment of the general subject, see Wallach's *Interpretation of Diagnostic Tests* [36]. The numbers in parentheses indicate normal ranges for these tests.

    A. Sodium (136–145 mEq/L)

        Increase: dehydration.

        Decrease: CHF, diuretic use, SIADH.

        Note:

            1. Hyperlipidemia and hyperglycemia are causes of spurious hyponatremia.

Nothing is more important to the care of the patient than the personal attention of a competent and conscientious physician. There is no substitute for the information a physician can obtain from a careful history and physical examination. This information should guide all diagnostic and therapeutic efforts. Without it, laboratory tests cannot be used effectively, therapeutic plans lack direction, and serious errors in management are likely to occur. The greatest mistake in the practice of internal medicine these days is the tendency to let indiscriminate laboratory testing and diagnostic procedures replace the common sense of the doctor. **Arnold S. Relman, M.D.**

2. Most hyponatremia is secondary to free water retention (in excess of retained sodium) rather than to sodium loss.

B. Potassium (3.5–5.2 mEq/L)

Increase: renal failure, acidosis, iatrogenic, mineralocorticoid deficiency.

Decrease: metabolic alkalosis, diuretic use, mineralocorticoid excess.

Note:

1. RBC hemolysis in blood sample acquisition can spuriously increase serum potassium.

2. Thrombocytosis spuriously elevates serum potassium.

3. Alterations in serum potassium may produce ECG changes (see Chap. 7, Part A, **III.E**).

C. Chloride (96–108 mEq/L)

Increase: dehydration, non-anion gap metabolic acidosis.

Decrease: diuretic use, CHF, SIADH, compensated respiratory acidosis, excessive emesis.

Note:

1. Hypochloremia is the most common cause of metabolic alkalosis.

2. The laboratory method for measuring chloride is a nonspecific test for halides; hence, bromides and iodides may spuriously elevate serum chloride.

D. Bicarbonate (24–30 mEq/L)

Increase: dehydration ("concentration alkalosis"), compensated respiratory acidosis.

Decrease: metabolic acidosis, compensated respiratory alkalosis.

E. Anion gap (10–12 mEq). The anion gap represents unmeasured anions, and is calculated as the difference in milliequivalents between serum sodium and the sum of serum chloride and bicarbonate.

Increase: renal failure, lactic acidosis, ketoacidosis, salicylate toxicity, ethylene glycol ingestion, methanol ingestion.

Decrease: multiple myeloma, bromide ingestion, polycythemia vera, DIC, pregnancy.

Note:

1. Use of the anion gap helps to distinguish two types of metabolic acidosis, i.e., hyperchloremic metabolic acidosis (that type associated with a *normal* anion gap) and high anion gap metabolic acidosis.

2. Note that some people define the anion gap as the difference in milliequivalents between the sum of sodium *and potassium* (rather than sodium alone), and the sum of chloride and bicarbonate; from a practical standpoint, either method may be used.

F. BUN (6–26 mg/dl)

Increase: renal failure of all types, accelerated protein catabolism (e.g., GI bleed), dehydration.

Decrease: liver damage, protein deficiency states.

G. Creatinine (0.7–1.7 mg/dl)

Increase: renal failure, muscle disease, increased muscle mass.

Decrease: rarely clinically significant.

Note:

1. Creatinine is a more specific indicator of renal disease than BUN.

2. The BUN-creatinine ratio is sometimes helpful in distinguishing prerenal azotemia (>20) from intrinsic renal disease producing azotemia (<20) (see Chap. 14, **IV**).

3. Hemodialysis of patients with CRF usually normalizes BUN: creatinine, however, may not change at all with dialysis.

H. Glucose (65–110 mg/dl)

Increase: diabetes mellitus, pregnancy, stress, pancreatic disease.

Decrease: reactive hypoglycemia, pancreatic islet cell tumors, starvation, liver disease.

Note: Measuring the fasting blood sugar (FBS) is the best method short of a formal oral glucose tolerance test to document diabetes mellitus.

I. Calcium (9.0–11.0 mg/dl)

Increase: malignancies, primary hyperparathyroidism.

Decrease: hypoparathyroidism, CRF, malabsorption syndromes, vitamin D deficiency, hypoalbuminemia.

Note:

1. Free ionized calcium is the physiologically important form of the cation; hence, correction must be made for the concentration of the major calcium-binding protein, albumin. (Correction = 0.8 mg/1.0 mg change in albumin.)

2. Changes in serum calcium are reflected in the ECG: an increase in calcium shortens the Q-T interval while a decrease in serum calcium lengthens the Q-T interval.

J. Phosphorus (2.5–4.2 mg/dl)

Increase: CRF, hypoparathyroidism.

Decrease: alcoholism, nutritional deficiency states.

Note: Hypophosphatemia can decrease myocardial contractility and effective tissue oxygenation (through decreased production of 2,3-DPG).

K. Albumin (3.5–5.5 gm/dl)

Increase: rarely clinically significant.

Decrease: chronic disease, nutritional deficiency states, protein-losing enteropathy.

L. Total protein (6.0–8.5 gm/dl)

Increase: multiple myeloma.

Decrease: chronic disease, protein-losing enteropathy.

Note: The difference between the levels of total protein and albumin is the amount of globulin.

M. Amylase (5–75 IU/L)

Increase: pancreatitis, mumps, parotitis, duodenal ulcer, ectopic pregnancy, diabetic ketoacidosis, biliary tract disease, peritonitis, macroamylasemia.

Decrease: pancreatic destruction.

Note:

1. Almost any intraabdominal process can elevate serum amylase.

    2. Salivary gland amylase and pancreatic amylase are different isozymes, and can be distinguished by electrophoretic analysis.

    3. The amylase-to-creatinine clearance ratio may be useful in distinguishing macroamylasemia (<1%) and other causes of ↑ amylase from pancreatitis (>5%).

N. Uric acid (1.5–8.0 mg/dl)

Increase: gout, asymptomatic hyperuricemia, renal failure, cancer with rapid tumor cell turnover, thiazide diuretics.

Decrease: allopurinol use, uricosuric agent use, Hodgkin's disease, Wilson's disease, aspirin ingestion.

Note: The greatest acute risk of elevated uric acid is the development of uric acid nephropathy, particularly in patients receiving chemotherapy. This can be avoided by adequate hydration, allopurinol therapy, and urinary alkalinization.

O. Cholesterol (140–260 mg/dl)

Increase: hypercholesterolemia, hyperlipidemia, biliary tract obstruction, pancreatitis, hypothyroidism.

Decrease: starvation, chronic disease, hyperthyroidism.

Note:

    1. Cholesterol levels increase postprandially.

    2. Cholesterol levels increase immediately after a myocardial infarction.

    3. Recent studies have clearly implicated elevated serum cholesterol in cardiovascular morbidity and mortality.

    4. The Western diet has led to a "normal" range for cholesterol that is probably too high. In fact, truly normal serum cholesterol is probably approximately 200 mg/dl or less.

P. Bilirubin (0.2–1.2 mg/dl)

Increase: **direct (conjugated) hyperbilirubinemia** (biliary obstruction, hepatitis), **indirect (unconjugated) hyperbilirubinemia** (hemolysis, Gilbert's syndrome).

Decrease: rarely clinically significant.

Note: The most prevalent cause of mild, asymptomatic unconjugated hyperbilirubinemia is Gilbert's syndrome.

Q. Alkaline phosphatase (30–115 units/L)

Increase: biliary tract obstruction, bone disease (especially Paget's disease).

Decrease: rarely clinically significant.

Note: Heat fractionation helps distinguish alkaline phosphatase of hepatic origin from that of bone origin ("bone burns"). Electrophoretic analysis of isozymes is also available.

R. SGOT (0–41 units/L)

Increase: myocardial infarction, hepatocellular disease, CHF, muscle disease, hemolysis.

Decrease: rarely clinically significant.

Note:

    1. SGOT elevation occurs in a host of disparate diseases. To say that the source of an elevated SGOT is infarcting myocardium, for example, requires that you interpret the elevated SGOT in the context of other abnormal chemistries (e.g., an elevated CPK).

2. SGPT may be useful in distinguishing an elevated SGOT of hepatic origin from that of other sources.

3. Elevations of SGOT, SGPT, and LDH suggest hepatocellular disease, whereas elevations of alkaline phosphatase and bilirubin suggest obstructive liver disease.

S. LDH (60–230 units/L)

Increase: myocardial infarction, CHF, muscle disease, neoplasia, hemolysis.

Decrease: rarely clinically significant.

Note: There are five isozymes of LDH, which can be electrophoretically fractionated. This fractionation is useful in distinguishing LDH elevations of myocardial origin (isoenzymes I and II) from that of other sources. An $LDH_1 : LDH_2$ ratio $\geqslant 1$ may be used to help predict recent myocardial infarction (within the last 3–5 days).

T. CPK (female   50–60 I.U./L; male   50–180 I.U./L)

Increase: myocardial infarction, striated muscle necrosis, cerebrovascular accident, hypothyroidism.

Decrease: rarely clinically significant.

Note:

1. Isozyme fractionation of CPK produces three bands: MM (striated muscle), MB (cardiac muscle), and BB (brain).

2. The MB band is elevated in an acute myocardial infarction.

3. Other sources of MB band include tongue and diaphragm.

4. The BB band is elevated in cerebrovascular accidents only if the blood-brain barrier is interrupted.

5. CPK is increased in hypothyroidism and renal failure because of decreased renal clearance.

B   **Practical Points Concerning the
                                          Serum Chemistries**

I. Ordering serum chemistry tests

A. You can **estimate the cost** of routine serum tests by assuming that each test costs about $10.

B. At many hospitals, you can **order just one test,** even though tests are done as automated batteries. If all you really care about is the potassium concentration, try ordering just that test rather than a full electrolyte panel. Because lab tests are done as automated batteries, you can often call the lab and get results of lab tests not originally requested.

C. Learn to think of serum chemistry tests in **groups:**

   1. The electrolytes (K, Na, Cl, HCO_3).

   2. Kidney function tests (BUN, creatinine)—also helpful in assessing fluid status.

   3. Liver function tests (SGOT, SGPT, albumin, total protein, bilirubin, alkaline phosphatase).

   4. Acute myocardial infarction enzymes (CPK, SGOT, LDH).

   5. Metabolic bone disease tests (Ca, P, alkaline phosphatase).

D. Know the status of each lab test that you have ordered (i.e., keep track of whether it has been officially ordered, drawn, received in the lab, and finished). Know the results on patients you are following; remember that you may call the lab to find the results if they have not made it back to the floor. A big part of learning to be an effective and efficient clinical clerk is knowing how to keep track of the progress of your patient's work-up.

E. Note that the electrolytes, BUN, creatinine, and glucose are often recorded quickly using a "standardized" lattice pattern:

$$\begin{array}{c|c}
Na & Cl \\
\hline
K & HCO_3
\end{array} \underset{\diagdown creatinine}{\overset{\diagup BUN}{\text{---glucose}}}$$

II. Interpreting serum chemistry tests

A. While it is easy to learn a simple collection of common variations in serum chemistries and their causes, it is not very practical. Unfortunately, on the wards you usually will not be faced with an isolated abnormal lab value (except for alkaline phosphatase or glucose); more often you will be confronted with a group of abnormal values derived from all the tests done in your test battery. For this reason, learn to recognize **common clinical patterns of abnormal routine serum chemistries,** such as those shown below. Note that in these examples the combination of values helps suggest a more limited and directed diagnosis than would any single abnormal value.

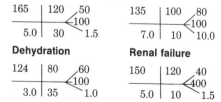

Dehydration   Renal failure

Excessive diuretic use Diabetic ketoacidosis

B. Remember that **lab error** is a common explanation for abnormal serum chemistry results. A wise clinician will try to repeat a lab test or confirm an abnormal result by some other test (e.g., an ECG can help confirm a high serum K) before acting on a lab result that does not seem appropriate for the clinical picture.

C. When prescribing any **medication,** keep in mind the lab tests that you would expect to be altered by the administration of the drug. Watch these test results carefully over the next few days, and use them to assess the efficacy or toxicity of your regimen. For example, diuretics commonly lead to hypokalemia.

7

Electrocardiography

A   Outline of Electrocardiography

I. **Indications for ordering an electrocardiogram.** Almost every patient you work up will need an ECG. In the patient with cardiac disease, the ECG will add to your growing understanding of the altered cardiovascular system, complementing the history and physical exam. In the noncardiac patient, the ECG screens for occult cardiac abnormalities and helps ensure the absence of acute disease. In both cardiac and noncardiac patients, the ECG provides a baseline picture of the heart and its conducting system to which future changes in cardiac status may be compared.

II. **Patterns analyzed in electrocardiographic analysis.** Basic analysis of the ECG includes:

   A. Rate and rhythm

   B. Axis

   C. P-R, QRS, and Q-T intervals

   D. QRS morphology

   E. S-T segment and T wave changes

   F. Comparison with previous tracings

III. **Analyzing and interpreting the electrocardiogram**

   A. Rate and rhythm

     1. Every ECG should be inspected to determine the heart's rate and rhythm. Rhythm is often not easily deciphered until the other basic patterns are considered. Decide first whether the ECG shows a normal sinus rhythm or an arrythmia. If a difficult arrhythmia is present, analyze basics **C–F (II)** as explained below (**C–G**), and then, armed with this information, return to sort out the arrhythmia (see Table 7-4).

     2. Rate mnemonics

       a. Regular rate. Recall that you can learn the rate quickly from the R-R interval. For a normal tracing (2.5 cm/sec or 5 large spaces marked by the heavier black line), an R-R interval of:

```
1 large box   = rate 300
2 large boxes = rate 150
3 large boxes = rate 100
4 large boxes = rate  75
5 large boxes = rate  60
6 large boxes = rate  50
```

Do not analyze the S-T segment and T wave until you have carefully scrutinized the QRS complex; pathologic alterations in the former can usually be explained by abnormalities in the latter.

Gilbert H. Mudge, Jr., M.D.

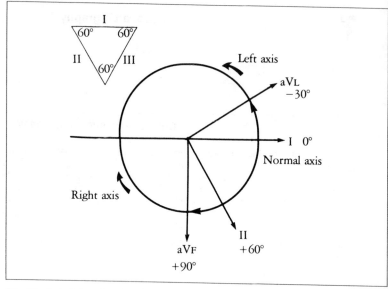

Fig. 7-1. Axis determination. Leads I, II, and III form a hypothetic equilateral triangle, with 60-degree angles as shown. Depolarization moving toward the left arm, parallel to lead I, is designated 0 degrees. Lead aVF, perpendicular to I, is thus labeled 90 degrees, and II is designated 60 degrees. Since aVL is perpendicular to II, forming a 90-degree angle, it is designated −30 degrees. (Reprinted with permission from G. H. Mudge, Jr., *Manual of Electrocardiography*. Boston: Little, Brown, 1981.)

- **b. Irregular or slow rate.** Note the small black marks at the very top of the ECG paper. At normal chart speed, these marks fall 3 seconds apart. Therefore, to find the rate of an irregular or slow rhythm, count out the number of beats in 2 consecutive 3-second spaces and multiple × 10.

- **c.** Always **check the atrial and ventricular rates separately.** Usually they will be the same; if they are not, a second- or third-degree heart block may be present.

B. Axis. Determine the axis for every cardiogram you read. To do this quickly, look at limb leads I, II, and aVF, noting whether the major direction of the QRS complex's deflection is positive or negative. Now recall the axis diagrams shown in Fig. 7-1. There are only three possibilities for axis that you need consider (+ represents upright QRS complex; − represents negative QRS complex deflection):

Lead I	Lead II	Lead aVF	Axis
+	+	+	between 0 and 90 degrees (normal)
−	+	+	>90 degrees (right axis deviation)
+	−	−	<30 degrees (left axis deviation)

If right axis deviation (RAD) is present, you must exclude right ventricular hypertrophy (RVH). If left axis deviation (LAD) is present, you must consider that left anterior fascicular block (LAFB) or left ventricular hypertrophy (LVH) is present. **If the axis is normal, it does not contribute significantly to the differential diagnosis, unless it has changed significantly from prior tracings.**

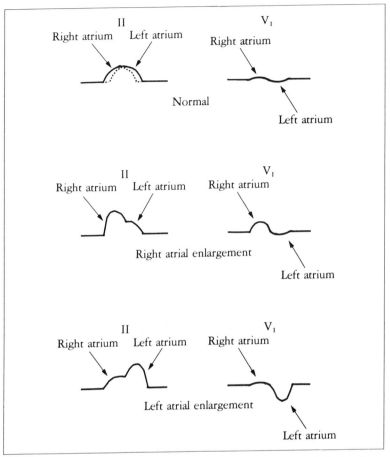

Fig. 7-2. P wave configuration. (Reprinted with permission from G. H. Mudge, Jr., *Manual of Electrocardiography*. Boston: Little, Brown, 1981.)

C. Intervals. Measure three intervals and record them:

Interval	Measure	Normal range	Physiologic correlate
P-R	Onset of P wave to onset of QRS complex	0.12–0.20 sec	Time spent between SA node depolarization to the initiation of ventricular depolarization, including conduction through the AV node
QRS	Onset to end of QRS	0.08–0.10 sec	Time required for the spread of the electrical impulse through the ventricular muscle
Q-T	Onset of QRS to end of T wave	Rate dependent but usually 0.32–0.40 sec	Time required for complete depolarization and repolarization

Table 7-1. Intraventricular conduction defects (IVCD)

IVCD	QRS duration	V_1 morphology	V_6 morphology
Right bundle branch block (RBBB)	≥0.12 sec	R′ in V_1	Deep S in V_6
Left bundle branch block (LBBB)*	≥0.12 sec	Wide S in V_1	Large R in V_6 often with jagged upstroke
Left anterior fascicular block (LAFB)	Diagnosis suggested by presence of axis ≤ $^-$30 degrees		
Left posterior fascicular block (LPFB)	Diagnosed by *newly* developed rightward shift in axis in the appropriate clinical setting (e.g., shift from +80 to +160 degrees in setting of an acute posterior MI or by extreme rightward axis)		

*In the presence of LBBB, no other conclusions may be read from the QRS morphology: hypertrophy, ischemia, and infarction are not reliably interpretable because of the abnormal pathway to ventricular depolarization.

1. **P-R.** If the P-R interval is >0.2 sec or is variable, a type of heart block is present. If it is <0.12 sec, this variant may be normal or it may be due either to a rhythm whose atrial focus is quite close to the AV node or to a preexcitation syndrome such as Wolff-Parkinson-White or Lown-Ganong-Levine syndromes.

2. **QRS.** The abnormal QRS duration is important in two instances. First, it will be prolonged in intraventricular conduction defects (IVCD), as outlined in Table 7-1. Second, in arrhythmia analysis, a wide QRS may indicate aberrant conduction of a supraventricular impulse or a ventricular ectopic focus (see the footnote to Table 7-4).

3. **Q-T.** The Q-T interval varies with heart rate. The corrected Q-T interval is $(Q-T)_C = Q-T \text{ (measured)} \div (R-R \text{ interval})^{1/2}$ and equals 0.42 sec. Usually the uncorrected Q-T interval is 0.32–0.40 seconds. Instances to be aware of that will alter the Q-T interval significantly include:

Quinidine	↑ QT	by increasing T wave duration
Hypocalcemia	↑ QT	by increasing length of S-T segment
Hypokalemia	↑ QT	by prolonging T wave with U wave formation
Hypercalcemia	↓ QT	by decreasing length of S-T segment

D. **QRS morphology.** The QRS complex is the most important configuration of the ECG. In addition to the duration of the QRS, which we have just considered, carefully analyze its morphology with respect to:

	Look for	Importance
General shape	Are there notches? Is the upstroke jagged or smooth?	Helpful in differential of IVCD
Height of R waves and depth of S waves	Especially in leads I, III, V_2, V_5	Helpful in determining presence of ventricular hypertrophy
Presence of Q waves	An initial downward deflection in the QRS, significant if > 0.4 sec (1 small box) or 25% height of associated R wave	A criterion for Q-wave myocardial infarction

E. **S-T segment and T wave changes.** One of the mistakes made by beginning electrocardiographers is to focus on the S-T and T wave changes without fully interpreting the QRS complex. The S-T segment and T wave should be analyzed once the QRS complex is evaluated. The S-T segment is most helpful in determining the presence of ischemic changes (Table 7-3). Remember that it may vary in normal individuals and is easily affected by drugs (especially digitalis) and electrolyte imbalance. Determine whether the ST segment is:

	Look for
Elevated or depressed	Elevation $\geq$ 1 mm or depression $\geq$ 0.5 mm
	Clinical correlates of ischemia
	Any drugs patient may be taking
T wave relation to S-T segment	Elevated S-T segment with T wave incorporated into S-T elevation suggestive of ischemia
	T wave that remains discernible from S-T segment elevation more consisent with normal variant (early repolarization)

The T wave is often a labile entity and changes in its morphology can be difficult to interpret. However, the presence of T wave inversion is often associated with three clinical situations: ischemia, digitalis, and *strain* (a pattern associated with ventricular hypertrophy). Determine whether the t wave is:

	Look for
Upright or inverted	Changes in leads I, II, and V_4-V_6, where T waves usually upright
Peaked or flattened	T waves peaking in the presence of $\uparrow K^+$
	T waves flattening as $K^+ \downarrow$ below normal range
	T waves altering their morphology as ischemic damage to the myocardium occurs

F. Arrhythmias. All of the information collected so far may be put to use in the analysis of arrhythmias. Table 7-4 elaborates on each arrhythmia and will be a useful supplement in your analysis.

A brief word first about **carotid sinus pressure (CSP),** a useful technique that employs the physiologic response of increased vagal tone to the AV node by stimulating the afferent limb of the carotid reflex. Two warnings should always be remembered. First, it is important to avoid CSP in patients who have a history of TIA or stroke or who have known carotid disease on exam. Second, this technique is not without complications even if you are cautious, and *must* be done in the presence of an experienced house officer with ECG monitoring.

Although the teaching of arrhythmia analysis is beyond the scope of this chapter, you can move a long way toward diagnosis by making this crucial distinction first: **is the rhythm in question regular or irregular?** Note the following diagnostic possibilities for these categories.

Regular rhythm	**Irregular rhythm**
Sinus tachycardia	Multifocal atrial tachycardia (MAT)
Paroxysmal atrial tachycardia (PAT)	Atrial fibrillation
PAT with block	Regular rhythm with variable block
Atrial flutter	
Ventricular tachycardia	

Once you have determined the category in which the rhythm in question belongs, there are several ways to analyze the rhythm further. For instance, the response to carotid sinus pressure, the P wave morphology, and the QRS morphology may all be helpful. Further information regarding the analysis of each arrhythmia is listed in Table 7-4.

Table 7-2. Quick checklist for the ECG

1. **Rate** (bradycardia? tachycardia? regular or irregular?)
2. **Axis** (RAD? LAD?)
3. **P wave morphology** (constant? saw-toothed? notched?)
4. **P-R interval** (<0.12? 0.12–0.20? >0.20?)
5. **QRS interval** (0.08–0.10? >0.10?)
6. **Q-T interval** (within range 0.32–0.40?)
7. **QRS morphology** (shape? height? depth? Q waves?)
8. **S-T segment** (elevated or depressed?)
9. **T wave** (upright or inverted? peaked or flattened?)
10. **Rhythm**
    a. Regular or irregular
    b. P/QRS relationship (1 : 1? extra P waves? extra QRS?)
    c. Reconsider P wave and QRS morphologies
11. **Previous tracing** (change in any lead? How recent?)

G. **Comparison with previous tracings.** It is important to compare the admitting ECG with previous tracings on record. The six basics of ECG analysis mentioned in sec. II (see also Table 7-2) should be compared in detail, and changes noted in the write-up. If there is no significant change, that fact should be specifically mentioned.

Table 7-3. ECG criteria for atrial abnormalities and ventricular hypertrophy

	P wave morphology		Major limb lead	Major precordial criteria	S-T and T wave changes
	II	V_2			
Left atrial abnormality (LAA)	See Fig. 7-2	See Fig. 7-2	—	—	None.
Right atrial abnormality (RAA)	See Fig. 7-2	See Fig. 7-2	—	—	None.
LVH (with or without strain)	—	—	R in I + S in III ≥ 20 mm	R in V_5 or V_6 + S in V_1 or V_2 ≥ 35 mm	S-T segment unchanged, T wave may be taller (without strain). S-T segment depressed, T wave inverted in leads V_4–V_6 (with strain).
RVH (with or without strain)	R/S ratio ≥ 1.0 in V_1 R/S ratio ≤ 1.0 in V_6		Right axis deviation (≥ + 90 degrees)	—	S-T segment unchanged, T wave may be taller (without strain). S-T segment depressed, T wave inverted in leads V_1, V_2 (with strain).

Table 7-4. Arrhythmias

Rhythms	Atrial rate	Ventricular rate	P wave morphology	CSP response	QRS morphology	Clinical points
Regular rhythms						
Sinus bradycardia	<60	<60	Normal	(Not used)	Normal	Often normal variant, especially in athletes.
						May accompany obstructive jaundice with ↑ serum bilirubin; ↑ intracranial pressure; digitalis; or acute inferior MIs.
						Most common cause at present is probably use of beta blocking drugs.
Sinus tachycardia	>100	>100	Normal	Gradual slowing; change to tachycardia when CSP released	Normal	Especially associated with fever, infections, hemorrhage, hyperthyroidism.

Paroxysmal atrial tachycardia	140–220	Usually obscured by preceding T wave Theoretically abnormal (focus other than SA node)	No change or abrupt termination of arrhythmia	Normal	May see S-T segment depression associated with PAT.
PAT with block	140–220	Fixed fraction of the atrial rate (e.g., 1/2)	Abnormal morphology	No change or ↑ in degree of block (e.g., from 1/2 to 1/4)	Normal	May indicate digitalis toxicity

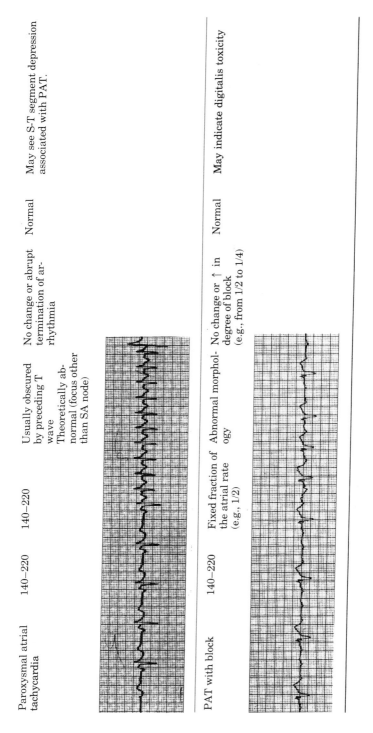

Table 7-4 (Continued)

Rhythms	Atrial rate	Ventricular rate	P wave morphology	CSP response	QRS morphology	Clinical points
Atrial flutter	220–320 (300–320 most common)	Fixed fraction of atrial rate (e.g., 1/2 or 1/4, so called 2:1 or 4:1 block)	Saw-toothed "Flutter" waves	Usually no change or ↑ in block	Normal	Look for flutter waves in II, III, aVf, V₁, and V₂.
Junctional tachycardia	>75	>75	None often; may be present in close proximity to QRS (either preceding or following); see Clinical points	No change or termination	Normal	Must exclude digitalis toxicity. Look for inverted P waves (from retrograde conduction) in II, III, and aVf. P waves may arrive at atria after QRS is inscribed and thus follow QRS on ECG.

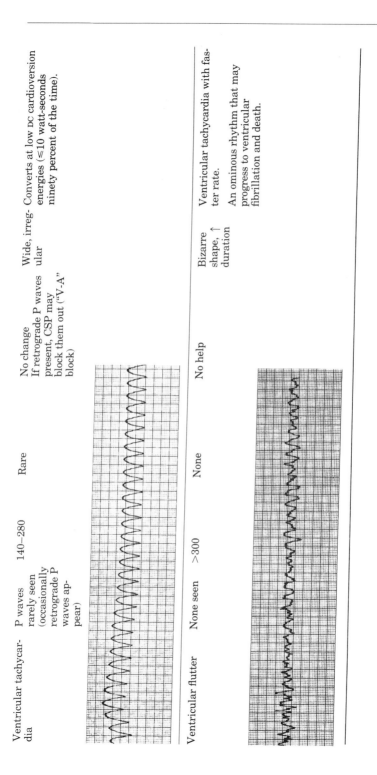

	P waves	Rate		CSP response	QRS	Comments
Ventricular tachycardia	P waves rarely seen (occasionally retrograde P waves appear)	140–280	Rare	No change. If retrograde P waves present, CSP may block them out ("V-A" block)	Wide, irregular	Converts at low DC cardioversion energies (≤10 watt-seconds ninety percent of the time).
Ventricular flutter	None seen	>300	None	No help	Bizarre shape, ↑ duration	Ventricular tachycardia with faster rate. An ominous rhythm that may progress to ventricular fibrillation and death.

Table 7-4 (Continued)

Rhythms	Atrial rate	Ventricular rate	P wave morphology	CSP response	QRS morphology	Clinical points
Irregular rhythms						
Multifocal atrial tachycardia (MAT)	>100	>100	≥3 different P wave morphologies	No change or transient slowing	Normal	Present in patients with COPD or pulmonary processes. Often must treat the primary process (not the arrhythmia).
Atrial fibrillation	None seen (flat or undulating baseline between Q waves)	40–300 (variable)	None	Usually no change; occasionally ↑ block	Normal	May be confused with atrial flutter. Classically associated with mitral stenosis and chronic mitral regurgitation; also present in CHF and coronary artery disease.

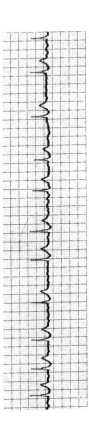

| Regular rhythm with variable block (not pictured) | 140–220 | Varying fraction of atrial rate (e.g., 2 : 1 block alternating with 4 : 1 block) | Abnormal | See PAT with block and Atrial flutter above | Normal | This is **not an irregularly irregular rhythm** like atrial fibrillation. |

Note: A widened QRS may be due to either (1) conduction of an impulse that originates in the atria but encounters refractory conduction tissue in the ventricular His-Purkinje system (**aberrant conduction**) or (2) an impulse that originates in ventricular tissue (**ventricular ectopic activity** [VEA]). In either case the widened QRS is due to electrical spread **directly** through ventricular muscle (outside the conducting system). Both mechanisms will lead to QRS interval prolongation, and making the distinction between them is often difficult. At this point it is sufficient to know that these two possibilities exist.

B

Practical Points Concerning Electrocardiography

I. Performing the electrocardiographic test

A. Within the first few weeks of your clinical rotations, learn how to perform a **12-lead ECG.** The key here is to aim for consistency in lead placement and a flat baseline. Remember to obtain a rhythm strip. The rhythm strip is usually done with lead V_2.

B. Realize that performing the ECG is a skill you will acquire with time; it is by no means necessary to your early success on the wards.

II. Patterns analyzed in electrocardiographic analysis

A. It is important to become comfortable enough with ECGs to be able to peruse them quickly and to detect abnormal features. The key task at this point is to pay attention to the basics of analysis described in Part A, sec. **II,** and to begin to train yourself to **recognize patterns,** i.e., to "eyeball" the tracing, first seeing the forest for the trees and then delving into the details of the tracing.

B. It is crucial to analyze the ECG within the **clinical setting.** This point may seem trivial, but it is in fact the most important consideration in ECG interpretation; the ECG has meaning for you as a clinician only in the context of the patient for whom you are caring.

III. Analyzing and interpreting the electrocardiogram

A. In preparation for learning ECG analysis, refamiliarize yourself with the anatomy and physiology of the **His-Purkinje system.** Also relearn the course and distribution of the **coronary arteries** if you have forgotten them.

B. Review a normal 12-lead ECG with particular attention to limb lead II and precordial lead V_2. Analyze the normal tracing step-by-step in the manner detailed in Part A, sec. **III** as a "warm-up" for the wards.

8

Chest Radiology

A

Annotated Outline of Chest Radiology

I. **Indications for ordering chest roentgenographs.** Chest radiology now occupies such an important place in the work-up of pulmonary, cardiovascular, and systemic problems that the chest roentgenograph or chest x-ray (CXR) has almost become an extension of the physical exam. There are many indications for ordering a chest film series, which routinely includes both posteroanterior (PA) and lateral views:

A. **Admission** chest x-rays are a standard part of the admission test battery at virtually all hospitals.

B. **Sepsis and fever** work-ups almost always include a chest x-ray, even if there are no obvious respiratory symptoms.

C. **Cardiovascular** pathologic processes are often accompanied by changes in the cardiac silhouette, the appearance of the great vessels, or the pattern of pulmonary vascular distribution.

D. **Pulmonary disease** processes as diverse as infection and neoplasm may be indistinguishable on the basis of the physical exam, and the CXR interpreted in the context of the clinical history is often the *sine qua non* of pulmonary diagnosis.

E. **Chest pain**, whenever thought to be due to musculoskeletal processes, routinely nvolves a chest x-ray as part of the diagnostic work-up. The CXR is especially

---

Acute pulmonary edema, in association with relatively *normal heart size*, develops in a number of specific clinical settings. Among these are:

Acute myocardial infarction
Acute glomerulonephritis
Fluid overload
Mitral stenosis
Drug sensitivity
Pregnancy with toxemia
Irritant gas inhalation
Trauma
Drowning
Exercise at high altitude
Heroin intoxication

Herbert Abrams, M.D.

One frequently sees on radiological reports, "The bones are *demineralized*." The term *demineralization* is used to refer to decreased bone mass, such as is seen frequently in the thoracic and lumbar spine of elderly women, as a manifestation of osteoporosis. There is no active demineralization, however, in the sense that decreased radiodensity is not due to the removal of the inorganic mineral phase from the bone matrix. *Decreased bone intensity* (a better term) results from removal of mineral *and* matrix in the process of remodelling with insufficient deposition of new bone to compensate for the losses from resorption.

S. M. Krane, M.D.

A coin lesion on the chest x-ray of an individual over the age of 40 with a history of smoking is carcinoma of the lung until proven otherwise.

Homayoun Kazemi, M.D.

indicated in patients with "atypical chest pain" syndromes, where one must decide between cardiovascular or noncardiovascular etiologies.

F. Systemic diseases often result in roentgenologic changes that, while rarely pathognomonic, are useful in diagnosis.

G. All of the pathologic processes mentioned in **B–F** can be followed with **serial chest x-ray studies,** although the radiologic picture may "lag behind" the clinical exam as a process resolves.

H. Interventional procedures such as thoracenteses and central line placements are often concluded with a chest x-ray to assess the efficacy (e.g., What is the position of a central line?) and rule out complications (e.g., Is there a pneumothorax?) of the procedure.

II. General approach to chest x-ray interpretation. Unlike many lab tests that can be successfully interpreted without any knowledge of the actual test methodology, the interpretation of all radiologic studies requires that the interpreter understand some basic radiologic principles. Most of these principles are intuitively obvious and follow from the concept that roentgenographs are actually **transilluminations of body structures,** similar to the transillumination of the cheek produced with a flashlight when one is investigating an oral lesion.

A. Radiologic densities and images. *The x-ray is a two-dimensional composite shadow produced by transmission of x-ray photons through three-dimensional structures* differing in ability to attenuate these photons. It gives two types of information: shape and density. There are several important corollaries to this concept.

    1. All shapes except a sphere will show dramatic changes in their **shadow profiles** depending on how the objects are positioned and rotated in front of the x-ray beam. Conversely, an object that looks circular on both the PA and lateral views is almost certainly spherical.

    2. An object will have a distinct **silhouette border** only if it differs significantly in density from the objects around it (the *silhouette sign*; see **III. A.2**). For the purposes of this chapter, there are **four basic densities:** (a) air, (b) fat, (c) tissue-fluid, and (d) bone. Because it is the most dense, bone will cause high levels of photon attenuation (and hence low photon transmission) and will appear to be the whitest on the x-ray. Conversely, the air in the lungs will allow high photon transmission and will show up as black or dark gray.

    3. A single image on the x-ray may involve the superimposition of multiple shadows. One must learn to use the PA and lateral views together in order to dissect composite shadows into shapes of individual objects.

B. Systematic roentgenographic interpretation. Like the physical exam, x-ray interpretation is best done in a systematic way, following the same sequence of analysis every time. Although the more experienced interpreter may "gestalt" a film, making an almost instant diagnosis after observing the integrated pattern for a few seconds (much like the snap diagnosis that an experienced clinician may be able to make), the novice radiologist should choose a certain sequence of analysis and stick to it. One useful sequence is to begin with the least prominent information on the film and gradually move toward the most prominent findings. Such an analysis sequence might be (1) introductory background information, (2) bones, (3) pulmonary vasculature, (4) pulmonary parenchyma and lung fields, and (5) cardiac silhouette and mediastinum.

These areas are discussed below. Fig. 8-1 is a reproduction of a normal PA and lateral chest x-ray with diagrams of the heart and great vessels superimposed to indicate their position.

    1. Introductory background information. Much information about the context of an x-ray study can be found on the film or the film folder. Always check

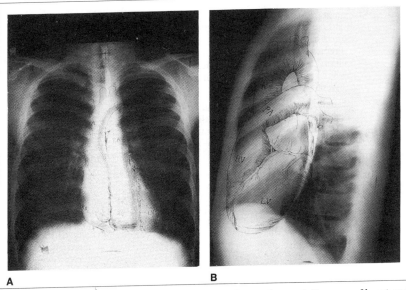

Fig. 8-1. CXR patterns of normal subject with superimposed diagrams of heart and great vessels. **A.** PA view. **B.** Lateral view.

this information first in order to ensure that you are looking at the correct CXR and understand the technique of the study. In particular, note:

a. **Patient name and number.** Films are often placed in the wrong file.

b. **Date of study.** Check the film itself, not just the envelope.

c. **Posteroanterior (PA) or anteroposterior (AP) projection.** Standard films are PA, while portable films are AP. AP views make the heart appear enlarged, and thus make true cardiac size difficult to assess.

d. **Supine or upright patient position.** Check stomach bubble position. Supine position causes increased prominence of pulmonary vasculature.

e. **Patient rotation.** Check the clavicles for symmetry. If the patient is rotated the film will be harder to interpret and to compare with other studies.

f. **Film penetration.** An underpenetrated film makes pulmonary vasculature more prominent.

g. **Dates of previous CXR studies.** Are old films available for comparison?

2. **Bone radiology in the chest x-ray.** Most CXR studies are not ordered to investigate the thoracic bones, but it is important to make a habit of looking at the bones every time you analyze a CXR both because the bones themselves may provide valuable diagnostic information about a patient's condition (especially in cases of systemic disease) and because the bones provide a kind of grid coordinate system, which will be useful in the identification, comparison, and description of the soft tissue.

An investigation of the bones often begins with the clavicles, whose symmetry allows an assessment of patient rotation, then proceeds to the shoulders, where one checks the appearance and relationships of the various elements of the joint and the general symmetry of the two shoulder joints. Although an appreciation for the texture and the limits of normal appearance of the skeletal system is difficult to acquire, the novice may make many diagnoses by paying special attention to any cortical breaks, fissures, "moth-eaten" areas, or areas that seem to have increased or decreased radiolucency when compared to the other bones and to the mirror image area on the other side of the body.

Finally, every rib may be individually located, mentally numbered, and visually inspected throughout the length of its spiral course. Once again, the clinical history is of paramount importance. A patient complaining of localized chest pain should have a very careful CXR rib analysis to rule out skeletal pathology, while the asymptomatic patient needs only a quick scan.

3. **Pulmonary vasculature.** One of the most important clinical questions encountered in chest radiology is whether or not the patient is in congestive heart failure (CHF). Although the pulmonary vascular pattern is useful in assessing other types of cardiopulmonary pathology, it is in the clinical setting of heart failure that the novice radiologist will most often be concerned with these patterns. In addition to the appearance of the heart itself, three features of the pulmonary vasculature appearance are important in making this diagnosis: (a) the pattern of vascular prominence and redistribution, (b) the existence of pulmonary edema, and (c) the finding of pleural effusion.

a. **Vascular patterns.** The vasculature is most prominent in the medial lower lung (75% of total perfusion is normally to the lower lobes due to the mass of lung parenchyma and gravitational effects).

The ratio of upper to lower vasculature is approximately 1 : 3 in the normal CXR. Vascular prominence can represent engorgement of arteries, veins, lymphatics, or all three. In general, pulmonary arteries run vertically, while pulmonary veins empty lower and course horizontally. Lymphatics are normally not visible. Although it is often difficult to decide between the arteries and veins on the basis of the x-ray alone, it is useful to remember that the back-up or regurgitation of blood from the left ventricle to the lungs (c/w mitral stenosis, CHF, MI, MR, etc.) will lead to venous prominence, while arterial engorgement will result from increased right-sided flow, as in left-to-right shunts (c/w patent ductus arteriosus, septal defects, etc.).

b. **Pulmonary edema.** Pulmonary edema is the result of pulmonic vascular congestion to the point where the oncotic pressure of the blood is no longer able to maintain the integrity of the vascular system. The resulting edema fluid is taken up by the pulmonary lymphatics, which increase in radiologic prominence due to the increased flow.

When the edema becomes severe, it is associated with **horizontal linear densities** known as *Kerley's lines*. Probably the most important of these are Kerley's B lines, which are assumed to represent engorgement of interlobular septa and are often observed in cases of CHF as well as tumor, fibrosis, and so forth (see Fig. 8-3).

c. **Pleural effusion.** The costophrenic angles should be sharp and free of fluid on the normal CXR. If the patient has made a good inspiratory effort, the diaphragm should be visible at the level of the rib 10–11.

Because pleural fluid collects in the costophrenic recess, in the upright patient it first fills up the deeper **posterior** part of the recess; practically, this means that the **lateral view** will show evidence of an effusion before the PA view. A caveat should be mentioned here: fluid may accumulate between the lung pleura and the diaphragm. In this case, the subpulmonic effusion may be difficult to distinguish from an elevated dia-

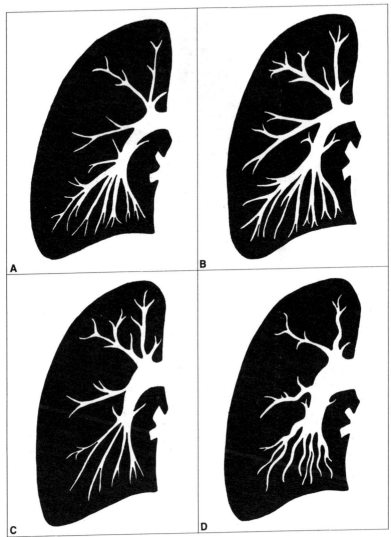

Fig. 8-2. Pulmonary vascular patterns in the right lung (PA film). In the normal lung, the majority of pulmonary perfusion is directed to the lower lobes, resulting in the CXR pattern seen in **(A)**. Generally increased vascular prominence without significant vascular redistribution is shown in **(B)**; this pattern represents the CXR of a patient with a high-output state such as left-to-right shunt, anemia, or pregnancy. Vascular redistribution as seen in congestive heart failure results in upper lobe engorgement and the pattern shown in **(C)**. **(D)** illustrates the central engorgement and peripheral vascular "pruning" seen in cases in which high peripheral pulmonary resistance due to lung disease results in pulmonary hypertension. (Modified from *The Merck Manual* [14th ed.]. Rahway, N.J.: Merck & Co., Inc., 1982.)

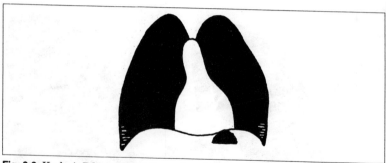

Fig. 8-3. Kerley's B lines. Small linear densities often found at the lung periphery, Kerley's B lines are assumed to represent engorgement of lymphatics due to pulmonary edema (see text).

phragm or a consolidated left lower lobe. Repeating the lung exam after looking at the x-ray often helps to resolve this confusion.

4. **Radiographic patterns.** The vascular shadows associated with normal and pathologic perfusion patterns are schematically illustrated in Fig. 8-2. Fig. 8-3 shows Kerley's B lines associated with pulmonary edema. While these diagrams are simplified and more obvious than the actual appearance of these findings on real chest x-rays, the student who begins by remembering these basic patterns and realizes that the pulmonary congestion found in congestive heart failure results in (a) venous engorgement with resultant increase in upper lobe vascular radiologic prominence, (b) pulmonary edema with Kerley's B lines, and (c) bilateral pleural effusions will already be able to comment usefully on many chest x-rays seen on a general medical service.

III. **Pulmonary parenchyma and lung field infiltrates.** While vascular problems present radiographically as linear densities, the roentgenographic changes suggesting disease in the pulmonary air-space compartment involve space-occupying, often "patchy" densities. Such findings are called **infiltrates,** and are associated with many types of disease processes, notably infections, neoplasms, and hemorrhage. The patient's clinical history and physical exam are very important in the interpretation of infiltrates; an infiltrate without a history of fever might suggest a hemorrhage or neoplasm, whereas a clinical history suggesting infection would place pneumonia much higher on the differential.

A. **Infiltrate localization.** The first step in analyzing an infiltrate is to attempt to determine exactly where it is. For the novice, there are three basic ways to locate an infiltrate:

1. Using the PA and lateral views together, an attempt is made to identify the three-dimensional location of the infiltrate. This is especially important in the analysis of small densities that may seem to represent coin lesions on the PA view but, when sought on the lateral, often turn out to signify either superficial structures (e.g., nipples, buttons) or collections of interlobular fluid (**pseudotumors**).

2. If an infiltrate is large enough to occupy a significant part of a lobe, it may result in the disappearance of the silhouette of an adjacent structure. This phenomenon is called the **silhouette sign,** and is actually nothing more than an application of the general principle that distinct outlines are visible on the x-ray only when there is a difference in density between adjacent structures. When lung tissue is replaced by blood, pus, or tumor, the radiographic outlines of the mediastinal or diaphragmatic organs superimposed on these infiltrated areas will disappear. By paying attention to exactly which outlines are obscured by the infiltrate, and by using both the PA and lateral

films, one can usually establish which lobes are involved, and gain insight into the etiology and extent of the infiltrate.

Fig. 8-4 illustrates the x-ray changes associated with consolidation in each of the pulmonary lobes. Note, for instance, that involvement of the right lower lobe, which is posterior, will lighten but will not totally obscure the right heart outline because the heart is anteriorly placed. By contrast, a right middle lobe infiltrate often obliterates the right side of the cardiac shadow.

3. The presence of some degree of **mediastinal shift** is a third key to deciding where a lesion is located. The mediastinum is normally a set of roughly midline structures. Note that these appear superimposed on the vertebral column in the normal PA film in Fig. 8-1. Consider especially the positions of the column of air in the trachea, the aortic arch, and the right heart border; these serve as reference points to the upper, middle, and lower mediastinum.

If the mediastinal structures appear to bow to one side, this may suggest either a *vacuum effect* caused by lung collapse, or a *mass effect* caused by neoplasm, exudate, or hyperinflation. Once again, the specific pulmonary lobes affected may be deduced from the mediastinal borders that are shifted. For instance, if only the right lower lobe is collapsed, the cardiac border will shift to the right while the trachea and the aortic arch may remain in their usual positions. The mediastinum will be shifted *toward* the side of lung collapse and *away* from the side of lung overexpansion (e.g., as in emphysematous change) and thoracic masses (e.g., as in pleural effusions, tumors). Shifts in the positions of the major and minor pulmonary fissures may be used in the same way. These are probably somewhat more revealing, although slightly more difficult to recognize.

B. **Infiltrate identification.** The radiologic differential diagnosis of pulmonary infiltrates is difficult and is dependent on the hints given by the clinical history. Often the most useful approach is to think in terms of broad categories of disease (e.g., infectious, neoplastic, collagen vascular, hemorrhagic) and then to use the clinical history to determine the most likely specific diagnosis. For instance, a right lower lobe infiltrate may suggest pneumonia, while the production of thick sputum with gram-positive diplococci would make the diagnosis of pneumococcal pneumonia virtually certain.

One very important question in the identification of a lung field density is whether the density is simply a collection of fluid located outside the alveoli or whether there is actual **consolidation** of the air spaces. A useful sign to look for is the presence of the **air bronchogram** pattern, which basically is nothing more than the air in the bronchial tree made visible by increased density of the surrounding structures. Normally, the bronchi are not well seen because there is not enough contrast in radiologic density; they consist of a tubelike arrangement of air spaces surrounded by a very thin wrapping of tissue. However, under conditions of lobar consolidation (due to tumor, pneumonia, etc.), the radiologic density surrounding these air spaces is much greater and the contrast makes the bronchial markings visible.

Table 8-1 summarizes some of the classic findings useful in the differential diagnosis of pulmonary infiltrate.

IV. **Cardiac silhouette.** An analysis of the cardiac silhouette on the chest roentgenograph extends the information acquired during the physical exam. For example, a soft S_3 coupled with an enlarged ventricle on CXR strongly suggests the possibility of congestive failure.

The key to interpretation of cardiovascular status as demonstrated on the CXR lies in the recognition of *specific chamber abnormalities*. Deciding that "the heart looks abnormal" is much less useful than deciding that there is dilatation of the left atrium, and straightening of the left heart border, suggestive of mitral valve disease.

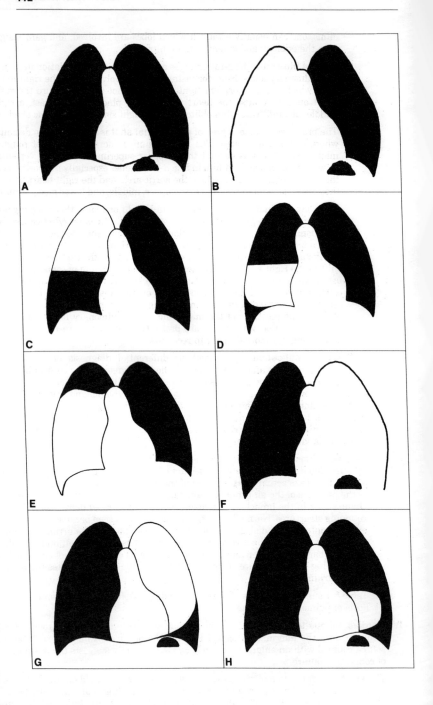

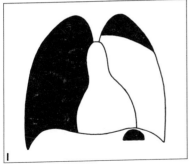

Fig. 8-4. CXR patterns produced by lobar consolidations such as those caused by pneumonia or tumor. Note the disappearance of various parts of the cardiac and diaphragmatic borders due to the increased density of the consolidated lung tissue. This loss of density contrast borders is called the *silhouette sign* (see text). **A.** Normal CXR. **B.** Total R lung consolidation with obliteration of the R heart border. **C.** R upper lobe consolidation. **D.** R middle lobe consolidation. **E.** R lower lobe consolidation. **F.** Total L lung consolidation with obliteration of the L heart border. **G.** L upper lobe lingular consolidation with disappearance of the L heart border. **H.** L upper lobe consolidation; L heart border still faintly visible due to air in lingula. **I.** L lower lobe consolidation; L heart border still faintly visible due to air in lingula. (Modified from L. Squire, *Fundamentals of Radiology* [rev. ed.]. Cambridge, Mass.: Harvard University Press, 1975.)

Table 8-1. Summary of roentgenologic findings associated with disease processes of various organ systems

Disease process	Roentgenographic findings
A. Cardiovascular*	
1. Atrial septal defect	RA and RV prominence with normal LA; prominent lung vascularity
2. Tricuspid regurgitation	RA enlargement; cardiac enlargement
3. Tricuspid stenosis	RA enlargement
4. Pulmonic regurgitation	No good CXR findings
5. Pulmonic stenosis	May be normal; otherwise, RV and outflow prominence; PA poststenotic dilatation
6. Pulmonary hypertension	RA and RV enlargement; prominent central pulmonary vessels near hilum; rapid tapering; avascular peripheral lung fields
7. Mitral regurgitation	LA and LV enlargement; mitral valve calcification; pulmonary congestion if chronic
8. Mitral stenosis	LA enlargement; prominent pulmonary venous system; mitral calcification; Kerley's B lines
9. Aortic regurgitation	LV enlargement; more prominent if chronic aortic dilatation
10. Aortic stenosis	Calcified aortic valve. LV enlargement; prominent ascending aorta
11. Hypertension	LV hypertrophy; prominent tortuous aorta
12. Congestive heart failure	LV enlargement and pulmonary congestion; Kerley's B lines
13. Constrictive pericarditis	Small or slightly enlarged heart; pericardial calcification
14. Coarctation of aorta	Notching of lower rib borders

Table 8-1 (Continued)

Disease process	Roentgenographic findings
B. Pulmonary infiltrates: infectious	
1. Viral pneumonia	Nodular infiltrate; diffuse involvement
2. Pneumococcal pneumonia	Lobar or bronchopneumonic infiltrates and consolidation; air bronchograms; pleural effusion
3. Tuberculosis	Apical infiltrate; parenchymal calcification
4. Granulomas (due to tuberculosis, histoplasmosis, coccidiodosis, etc.)	Fibrosis; calcifications; satellite densities
C. Neoplasms	
1. Bronchogenic carcinoma	Solitary lesions without calcifications
2. Bronchoalveolar cell cancer	Segmental distribution; can mimic infiltrate
3. Metastatic cancer	Often multiple lesions
4. Hodgkin's disease, lymphoma, leukemia	Parenchymal infiltrate; hilar node enlargement; mediastinal widening
D. Pulmonary	
1. Foreign body	Foreign body may be obvious on CXR; may cause "check valve" hyperinflation
2. Atelectasis	Plate-like densities
3. Bronchiectasis	Basilar patchy densities
4. Emphysema	Overexpanded lungs; low diaphragms; increased radiolucency of lungs; heart may seem small
5. Interstitial lung disease (due to inhalants, drugs, collagen vascular disease, etc.)	Diffuse infiltrate
6. Pneumothorax	Visceral pleural line visible on x-ray

*Cardiac enlargement is usually a late finding in cardiovascular diseases.

A. **Components of the cardiac silhouette.** The borders of the cardiac shadow can be decomposed into a series of nine overlapping arcs (Fig. 8-5). The systematic analysis of the cardiac shadow involves breaking the shadow down into these arcs and determining which, if any, are abnormal. Once the information in Fig. 8-5 is memorized, it becomes much easier to apply knowledge of cardiovascular pathophysiology to the interpretation of the chest film.

B. **Cardiothoracic ratio.** A specific example of the use of cardiac chamber appearance in radiologic diagnosis is the cardiothoracic ratio. This concept, illustrated in Fig. 8-6, is based on the rule of thumb that, in the PA exposure, the extreme right and left borders of the cardiac outline (segment A-B) should be no farther apart than one-half the width of the chest at its widest point (segment C-D). Because an enlarged left ventricle is most often the cause of an enlarged cardiothoracic ratio, this rule is most useful in the diagnosis of heart failure associated with ventricular dilatation or hypertrophy.

Fig. 8-7, a reproduction of the lateral CXR of a patient who has undergone triple valve replacement, clarifies the position of the cardiac valves and outflow tracts.

Table 8-1 summarizes some of the common CXR findings associated with specific cardiovascular problems.

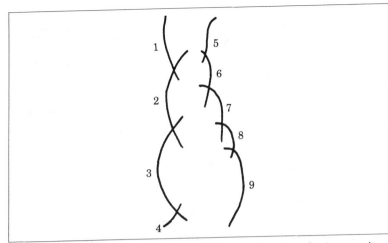

Fig. 8-5. The normal mediastinal profiles are all vascular and resolve into a series of nine intersecting arcs: (1) superior vena cava; (2) ascending aorta; (3) right atrium; (4) inferior vena cava and cardiac fat pad; (5) left subclavian vein and artery, left common carotid artery; (6) aortic arch; (7) pulmonary artery; (8) left atrium; (9) left ventricle. (Reprinted with permission from L. Squire, *Fundamentals of Radiology* [rev. ed.]. Cambridge, Mass.: Harvard University Press, 1975.)

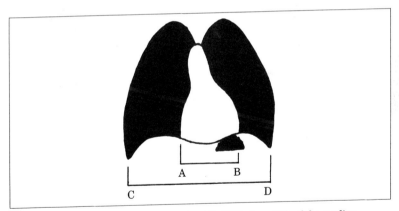

Fig. 8-6. Cardiothoracic ratio. In a routine PA CXR, the width of the cardiac shadow (segment A-B) should be no more than half the width of the thoracic cavity (segment C-D). This rule of thumb is rough and should be used together with an analysis of the cardiac chamber configuration to obtain a reasonable estimate of heart size (see text).

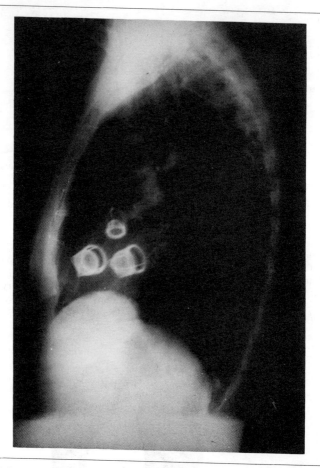

Fig. 8-7. Lateral CXR of patient who has undergone aortic, mitral, and tricuspid valve replacement demonstrating the position of these valves and their outflow tracts (compare with Fig. 8-1).

| **B** | **Practical Points Concerning Chest Radiology** |

I. Ordering the chest roentgenograph

A. The **requisition form** for a CXR usually includes a space for you to provide **clinical information** to be used in the radiologist's interpretation of the film. It is important that you provide the radiologist with two types of information:

1. The clinical history that relates to your **specific questions** (e.g., "55-year-old male with long smoking history and recent weight loss and chronic fever; rule out cancer.").

2. Clinical details relating to known **x-ray findings** that might otherwise confuse the radiologist (e.g., "Patient has history of pulmonary radiation treatment 2 years prior to admission.").

The better your clinical summary, the better your radiology reports will be.

B. Every radiology department has its own set of **protocols** for working up specific problems. It is worth your while to talk to a radiologist about the department's preferences (e.g., "Should a suspicious CXR be followed by plain lung tomography or by a CT scan of the chest?"). Try to use the radiologist as a diagnostic consultant as well as a film interpreter. In the process you will learn a lot of medicine.

II. General approach to chest x-ray interpretation

A. Before attempting to interpret chest x-rays, you should review the gross anatomy of the **thorax**, concentrating especially on:

1. The relations of the internal organs in the thorax, especially the mediastinal structures around the T_4 level (e.g., determine the relation of the heart to the tracheal bifurcation and the esophagus).

2. The exact position of the heart and its chambers in the thorax. Think about possible pathophysiologic changes in the shape of the heart. For instance, where on the cardiac margin would you see the protruding atrium in an instance of left atrial dilatation? What diseases might cause this change?

3. The lobes of the lungs and the approximate positions of the pulmonary fissures. Which fissures would you expect to see from the PA perspective? Which from the lateral?

B. Common sense principles are of the utmost importance in attempting to learn CXR interpretation. Keep the following general principles in mind:

1. With certain obvious exceptions, the human body is a bilaterally symmetric structure. Consequently, an area on one of the lungs that appears to demonstrate vascular prominence may be profitably compared to the mirror image area on the other lung (bearing in mind, of course, that the lungs themselves are not perfectly symmetric).

2. **Changes** in serial x-ray studies are of the utmost importance, especially if the changes occur around the time that the patient's clinical history changes. Try to review the patient's x-ray files to find when the films first began to deviate from normal. To develop the ability to recognize changes you will have to study many normal films and pay careful attention to serial films taken on your patients. For patients who receive a film daily, take the time every so often to compare that day's film to one taken a week earlier. Changes may be more obvious.

3. Although it is often a good teaching exercise to try to interpret an x-ray before you read the clinical history, you should always think about your patients' films in relation to their clinical conditions. Could you hear râles in the patient whose chest films suggest pulmonary edema? Was there the sudden onset of pleuritic pain or dyspnea just before the patient's films began to show a segmental lower lobe infiltrate consistent with a pulmonary embolus? You should constantly recheck old films as the clinical story evolves; often an old x-ray finding can be reinterpreted in light of new information. You should learn to use the x-rays to sharpen your physical examination skills; the **listen-look-listen** method (*listen* to the lungs; *look* at the x-ray; *listen* to the lungs again) is an excellent self-teaching device.

4. **Pathophysiologic processes** that are very different clinically may look very similar on the x-ray (for instance, bronchoalveolar cell carcinoma may appear identical on x-ray to lobar pneumonia). Therefore, the vocabulary with which you speak of and think about the roentgenograph should be that of radiologic appearance ("nodule," "opacity," "infiltrate") and not diagnosis ("tumor," "granuloma," "pneumonia"). First describe what you see; then attempt to interpret it in light of the facts of the case. The essence of radiology is shrewd pattern recognition coupled with a knowledge of radiologic differential diagnosis.

5. **Straight lines** usually belong in the province of physics, not biology. Differentiate between discrete lines, such as a fibrotic strand, and a straight interface, such as a pleural effusion. If you see an anomalous straight line cutting across a film, consider the possibility that it is caused by fluid collecting under the force of gravity or by something extrinsic to the thorax. Tilting the patient often causes a change in the fluid level, which may help in your interpretation. The gas-fluid interface in the stomach (*stomach bubble*) helps you decide if the patient was standing up or lying down when the film was taken.

6. **Displaced organs** and anatomic structures generally suggest that something is either pushing or pulling them out of normal position, even though the deforming agent or process may not be visible on the x-ray. (A 16-year-old girl with a history of Hodgkin's disease whose chest film shows progressively increased splaying of the carina would therefore be investigated carefully for possible relapse.)

III. **Chest x-ray interpretation.** As a medical student doing core clinical rotations, you will be confronted with two different scenarios during which you will be asked to interpret the CXR.

A. **Reviewing your patients' roentgenographs** before you have obtained an "official" intepretation from a radiologist should be a routine part of your work-up, just like looking at the urine sediment or interpreting the ECG. Though you may wish to consult a radiologist before deciding on further diagnostic or treatment plans, you should formulate your own opinion of the CXR findings before asking for an expert opinion. Moreover, radiologists are often excellent teachers and will spend much more time with a student who seems to have some idea of basic radiologic principles than with one who simply puts a CXR on the viewbox and asks, "Is this normal?" Table 8-2 is a quick checklist for the review of a CXR.

When presenting roentgenographs as part of formal case presentations, it is best to be systematic and complete. Many radiologists use the following algorithm:

1. Describe what you see in very general terms.

2. Describe the pertinent findings that you do **not** see.

3. Give the radiologic differential diagnosis.

4. Now use the clinical history to defend your top diagnosis or group of diagnoses.

5. Finally, suggest what further studies should be done to arrive at a definitive diagnosis.

An example of a formal CXR interpretation follows:

There is a patchy wedge-shaped density in the right lung field, best seen on the lateral view. The hemidiaphragms are flat and there is some linear scarring at the bases. The heart and great vessels appear normal. I do **not** see any evidence of pleural effusion, and there are no air bronchograms. The top differential diagnosis would be right middle lobe pneumonia superimposed on a picture of chronic bronchitis versus a tumor. The clinical history of acute onset cough and green sputum production favors the diagnosis of pneumonia, but in a man with 75 pack-year smoking history, a tumor must be vigorously excluded. The trial of antibiotics that you are presently undertaking will be informative. Bronchoscopy would probably be the next step in the evaluation of the infiltrate if no response to the antibiotic course is noted.

B. The **spot analysis** of a CXR is a frequent part of teaching rounds. A student will be asked to give an off-the-cuff analysis of a CXR that he or she has never seen before and knows nothing about. The best approach here is to be systematic. *Spend about 20 seconds looking at the CXR without saying anything.* If you want to, you can stall for time by saying something such as, "I would have to know a bit of clinical history before being able to make a reasonable statement." (You may not get it, but you can always ask.) The first determination you must make is the organ system or systems involved in the abnormality. Once you have decided on the **type of process** going on, you can then refine your statements by zeroing in on the **exact findings.** A typical student-level spot analysis might be, "These lung fields look congested. There is a moderate degree of pulmonary vascular redistribution bilaterally. I don't see any Kerley's B lines, but there is a small pleural effusion on the right, seen best in the lateral. The heart looks big and the profile suggests left ventricular dilatation. I don't see any infiltrates or bony lesions. Overall, I would call this a picture of moderate congestive heart failure."

Table 8-2. Quick checklist for the CXR

A. PA views

1. Clavicles (rotation?)

2. Bones (lesions?)

3. Breasts, soft tissue

4. Costophrenic angles (inspiratory effort? pleural effusion?)

5. Lung markings (engorgement? redistribution? hydrothorax or pneumothorax?)

6. Lung fields (coin lesions? consolidation? hilar adenopathy?)

7. Mediastinal shift

8. Cardiac shadow (cardiothoracic ratio? pericardial effusion?)

9. Specific cardiac chamber profiles (dilatation or hypertrophy? aortic profile?)

B. Lateral views

1. Right and left diaphragm outlines

2. Posterior sulci (pleural effusion?)

3. Thoracic vertebrae

4. Hilar markings

5. Trachea (air column position?)

6. Anterior and posterior clear spaces

7. Cardiac shadow (profile? specific chamber enlargement?)

Though detailed compilations of colorplates may be found in most comprehensive specialty texts, a smaller number of core illustrations is appropriate for an introductory manual. Colorplates A and B demonstrate the routine Gram stain procedure (see detailed explanation of these in the following paragraphs), and Colorplate C displays the characteristic Gram stain appearance of the most commonly encountered microorganisms. Colorplate D demonstrates the actual appearance of many of these organisms under 1,000 × (oil-immersion) magnification. They are identified in the table following the colorplates. Similarly, Colorplates E-I display some basic dermatologic lesions with which every student should be familiar.

Colorplate A. The Gram stain reaction is of primary importance in the morphologic and taxonomic classification of bacteria. A simplified, brief version is presented here. **The smear should be thin, air-dried, and gently heat-fixed.**

1. Flood the slide with **crystal violet**—10 seconds. (Wash with running tap water.)
2. Flood with **Gram's iodine** (brown)—10 seconds. (Wash with water.)
3. Carefully **decolorize with 95% ethanol or ethanol-acetone mixture** until the thinnest parts of the smear are colorless. (Wash with water.)
4. Flood with **safranin** (red)—10 seconds or longer if hard-to-see gram-negative organisms such as *Bacteroides* or *Haemophilus* are suspected.
5. **Results.** Organisms that retain the violet-iodine complex after washing in ethanol will stain **purple (gram-positive);** those that lose this complex will stain **red (gram-negative)** from the safranin counterstain. Although the mechanism of this reaction is not completely understood, a plausible explanation is that the cell walls of gram-positive bacteria contain less lipid than the cell walls of gram-negative organisms and therefore are less permeable to organic solvents. This enables gram-positive bacteria to retain the violet-iodine complex. In a properly executed Gram-stained smear, **cellular elements and most background material stain pink to red.**

Colorplate B. The clinician can quickly assess the adequacy of the Gram stain by comparing several different areas of the slide, using the oil-immersion lens. Granulocyte nuclei and gram-negative organisms in a thin area of the smear should stain red, and gram-positive organisms should stain purple (see # 3). Finding red bacteria near slightly purple (marginally decolorized) cellular elements in a thicker part of the smear can confirm that bona fide gram-negative organisms are present (see # 2) rather than over-decolorized gram-positive bacteria (see # 4). Fields wholly under-decolorized (see # 1) indicate only the presence of the bacteria but not necessarily their staining characteristics.

Prepare thin smear. Air-dry and heat-fix.

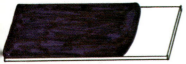

1. Flood with crystal violet 10 seconds. Rinse with tap water.

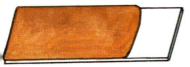

2. Flood with Gram's iodine 10 seconds. Rinse.

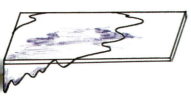

3. Critical step: Decolorize and rinse.

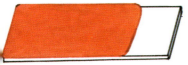

4. Flood with safranin counterstain 10 seconds or more. Rinse. Blot or air-dry.

A. Gram-stain method.

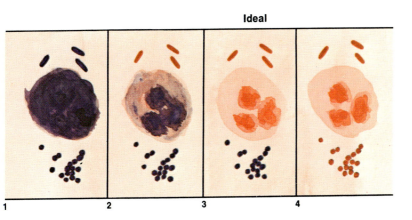

B. Variations possible on a Gram stain.

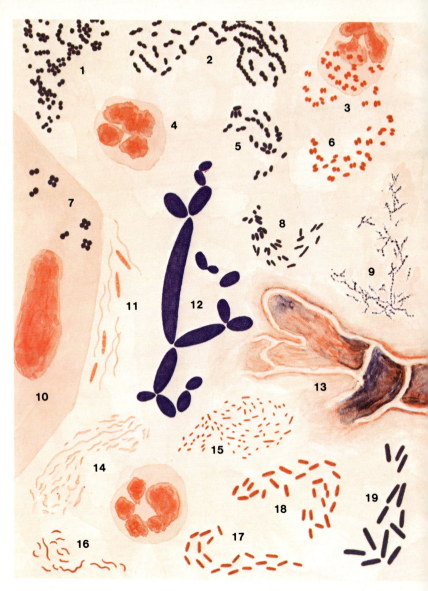

C. Morphology and Gram-stained characteristics of organisms frequently encountered in clinical specimens. Average-sized organisms, shown here in scale and as they appear under optimal conditions, are usually seen at 1,000× (oil-immersion lens).

1. *Staphylococcus*
2. *Streptococcus* and Pneumococcus
3. *Neisseria*
4. Polymorphonuclear leukocyte
5. *Listeria*
6. *Acinetobacter (Mima, Herellea)*
7. *Micrococcus*
8. *Corynebacterium* (diphtheroids)
9. *Nocardia* or *Actinomyces*
10. Epithelial cell
11. *Fusobacterium* and *Borrelia*
12. *Candida*
13. *Aspergillus* (higher fungi usually do not take up Gram stain)
14. *Bacteroides*
15. *Haemophilus* (and other often rare organisms such as *Pasteurella*)
16. *Vibrio*
17. *Pseudomonas*
18. Enterobacteriaceae (*Escherichia coli, Proteus, Salmonella,* etc.)
19. *Clostridium, Bacillus,* or *Lactobacillus*

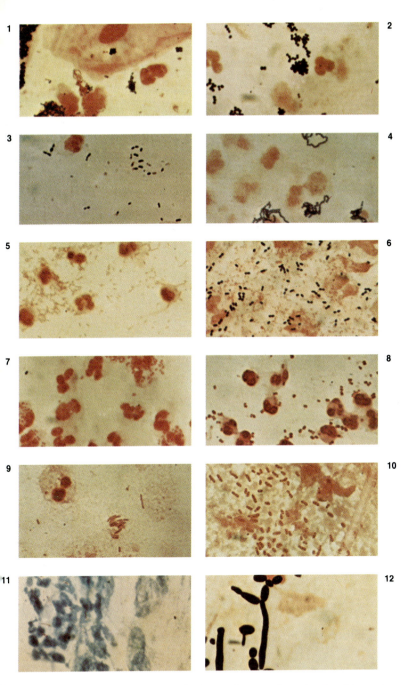

Ⅰ. Photomicrographs of various pathogens. All photographs were taken using the oil-immersion lens (×1,000) and are Gram-stained specimens, with the exception of number 11, which was stained by the Ziehl-Neelsen method. Descriptions of these organisms are given in the table following Colorplate Ⅰ.

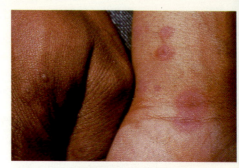

E. Erythema multiforme—iris (target) lesions.

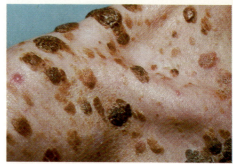

F. Seborrheic keratoses.

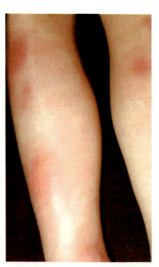

G. Erythema nodosum.

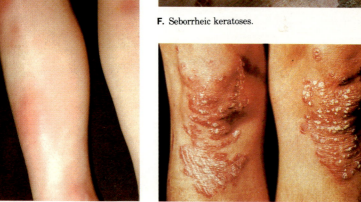

H. Psoriasis.

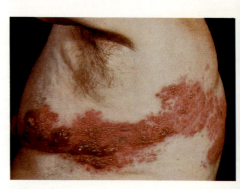

I. Herpes zoster.

Descriptions of the organisms in Colorplate D

Number	Specimen	Observation	Likely possibility	Culture report	Comment
1	Throat	Epithelial cell, gram-positive and gram-negative cocci, small gram-positive rods, thin gram-negative rods	Variety of organisms—normal throat flora	Normal throat flora	No inflammatory cells, wide variety of organisms. Specimen not indicative of infection.
2	Sputum	Gram-positive cocci in singles, pairs, and clusters; neutrophils	Staphylococcus	*Staphylococcus aureus*	Classic smear of staphylococcal pneumonia.
3	CSF	Gram-positive and gram-variable cocci in pairs and short chains; PMNs	Pneumococci or streptococci	Pneumococcus (*Streptococcus pneumoniae*)	Neutrophils are stained correctly; nearby organism is nicely gram-positive. Since only one kind of organism usually causes meningitis, and gram-positive organisms may become gram-negative with age, etc., it is likely that all these organisms are gram-positive cocci.
4	Knee joint fluid	Gram-positive cocci in long chains	Streptococci	Group A streptococcus (*Streptococcus pyogenes*)	Gram-positive cocci in very long chains, although conceivably pneumococci, are most likely to be streptococci.
5	CSF	Small gram-negative coccobacilli and rods	*Haemophilus*, remote chance of other small gram-negative organism such as *Pasteurella*	*Haemophilus influenzae*	Small gram-negative cocci, coccobacilli, and relatively slender rod forms are typical of *H. influenzae*.

Descriptions of the organisms in Colorplate D (Continued)

Number	Specimen	Observation	Likely possibility	Culture report	Comment
6	Sputum	Gram-positive cocci in pairs, small gram-negative coccobacilli, hints of neutrophils	Pneumococci, *Haemophilus*	Pneumococcus, *Haemophilus influenzae*	Sputum from patients with chronic bronchitis often contains *H. influenzae*—here, an active infection of pneumococci is superimposed. Gram-negative organisms can be especially hard to see in mixed infections. Always carefully examine the background!
7	Urethra	Gram-negative intracellular diplococci (GNID)	*Neisseria* spp.	Gonococcus (*Neisseria gonorrhoeae*)	Classic smear of gonococci—abundant intracellular organisms in many, but not all, PMNs. Although *Acinetobacter (Mima, Herellea)* organisms may be morphologically similar to *Neisseria*, they usually do not evoke such a neutrophil response and normally occur in a different clinical setting.
8	CSF	Gram-negative diplococci, neutrophils	*Neisseria*, remote chance *Acinetobacter*	Meningococcus (*Neisseria meningitidis*)	Classic *Neisseria*—note coffee-bean shape and snug "belly-to-belly" alignment, different from paired pneumococci, which do not have adjacent sides flattened. Organisms in CSF do not have to be intracellular to be considered significant.

9	Unspun urine	Gram-negative rods, neutrophil	*Escherichia coli*	Presence of one or more organisms per oil-immersion field of unspun urine indicates 10^5 or more bacteria per milliliter. Note that the enteric gram-negative rods tend to be larger and plumper than those of *H. influenzae*.
10	Sputum	Plump, beaded, gram-negative rods	*Klebsiella*	Although *Klebsiella* often appears as large, plump, beaded rods with a hint of capsule, it has no monopoly on these characteristics and need not exhibit them.
11	Sputum	Small red bacilli, many with granules (Ziehl-Neelsen stain)	*Mycobacterium tuberculosis*	Gram's stain typically revealed no organisms. Acid-fast stain obligatory.
12	Sputum	Budding yeasts with pseudohyphae	*Candida albicans*	Although budding yeast forms are indistinguishable from one another, abundant pseudohyphae in tissue suggest *Candida* spp.

Additional organism column entries: row 9 "Enteric gram-negative rod"; row 10 "Enteric gram-negative rod such as *Klebsiella*"; row 11 "Acid-fast bacilli"; row 12 "*Candida* spp."

Source: Adapted from P. Gardner and H. T. Provine, *Manual of Acute Bacterial Infections* (2nd ed.). Boston: Little, Brown, 1984. Pp. 183–190.

9   Arterial Blood Gas Determination

A   Annotated Outline of Arterial Blood Gas Determinations

I. **Indications for testing arterial blood gas.** The arterial blood gas (ABG) determination is a general test of cardiopulmonary function and acid-base status. Because a sample of arterial blood is somewhat difficult and painful to collect, this test is obtained only when there is a serious possibility of altered ventilatory status, hypoxemia, hypocapnia, hypercapnia, or a pH disturbance. Common clinical situations in which these disturbances are encountered include:

   A. Suspected **myocardial infarction** or **cardiac arrest.**

   B. **Respiratory distress** secondary to asthma or chronic obstructure pulmonary disease.

   C. **Stroke** with altered level of consciousness.

   D. **Right-to-left circulatory shunt.**

   E. **Suspected acid-base disturbance.**

   F. **Poisoning** or **trauma** with cardiopulmonary depression.

II. **Parts of the arterial blood gas determination.** Five results are commonly reported on an ABG determination:

   A. Partial pressure of oxygen (**PO_2**: normal 80–95 mm Hg).

   B. Oxygen saturation (**SaO_2:** normal 93–98%).

   C. Partial pressure of CO_2 (**PCO_2:** normal 36–43 mm Hg).

   D. CO_2 [HCO_3] content (**CO_2:** normal 20–30 mEq/L).

   E. Arterial pH (**pH**: normal 7.35–7.45).

   All of these tests are usually performed together by an automated analyzer.

III. **Intepreting the arterial blood gas determination.** Because the body has compensatory mechanisms to respond to acid-base disturbances (e.g., increasing exhalation of carbon dioxide in order to correct a metabolic acidosis), ABG values must be analyzed together to give a good indication of the true acid-base status of the patient.

Patients with decompensated congestive heart failure, cirrhosis with ascites, chronic renal or respiratory insufficiency, or other chronic disease states have often taken weeks or months to reach the point where they seek medical attention. The physician must avoid the error of attempting to correct the problem in a day. Overly aggressive efforts to achieve dry weight or normal electrolyte and acid-base status are fraught with hazard. The proper goal is to get the patient a little better each day, assessing progress in a time frame appropriate to the duration of the patient's illness.

Thomas W. Smith, M.D.

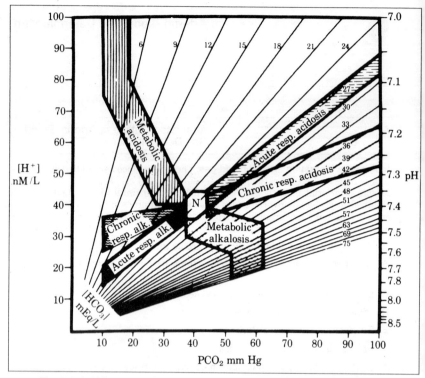

Fig. 9-1. Acid-base map showing the usual compensatory range of pH, PCO_2, and plasma HCO_3^- concentrations in simple acid-base disorders. Values on the vertical axis represent plasma H^+ concentration (left) in nanomoles per liter, or pH (right). Values on the horizontal axis represent PCO_2 in mm Hg. Diagonal lines are isopleths for the plasma HCO_3^- concentration in mEq/L. Clear area in the center of the graph is the range of normal. Note that the metabolic component (plasma HCO_3^- concentration) and the respiratory component (arterial blood PCO_2) of the acid-base equation always change in the same direction. (Reprinted by permission from M. Goldberg et al., Computer-based instruction and diagnosis of acid-base disorders: A systemic approach. *J.A.M.A.* 223:269, 1973. Copyright © 1973, American Medical Association.)

Fig. 9-1 is a nomogram that allows rapid systematic interpretation of ABG results (see its legend for further explanation).

IV. **Interpreting the arterial blood gas results.** Like most clinical lab tests, the ABGs are best approached systematically until the basics are mastered. The following sections outline a beginner's approach to the interpretation of acid-base disorders.

   A. **What is the pH?** If it is less than 7.35, you are dealing with an acidosis of some sort. If it is higher than 7.45, a form of alkalosis is present. Remember that a pH in the normal range (7.35–7.45) does not exclude an acid-base disorder since compensated or mixed disorders may have pH values within the normal range.

   B. **If an acidosis exists, is it primarily respiratory or metabolic?** To determine this, look at the PCO_2 and $[HCO_3]$.

1. **PCO$_2$ > 45 mm Hg** indicates a respiratory acidosis. Common etiologies include entities that can contribute to a buildup of CO_2, such as COPD, pneumonia, CNS depression, pulmonary edema, cardiopulmonary arrest, airway or chest wall injury, drugs, and neuromuscular disease. The [HCO$_3$] will be normal in the early stages of a simple respiratory acidosis, but will increase in chronic acidosis as the body tries to compensate for the high PCO$_2$.

2. **[HCO$_3$] < 22 mEq/L** indicates a metabolic acidosis involving a fall in the serum [HCO$_3$]. Common etiologies include diabetic and lactic acidoses (e.g., acute MI), diarrhea, dehydration, shock, toxins (e.g., aspirin), and iatrogenic causes, including NH_4Cl and acetazolamide administration. The PCO$_2$ will usually fall as the lungs attempt to correct the acidosis by blowing off CO_2 (the **Kussmaul respirations** of diabetic ketoacidosis).

   The key to the differential diagnosis of metabolic acidoses involves an analysis of the **anion gap** [Na − (Cl + HCo$_3$)] (see Chap. 6, Part A, **II.E**). Disorders such as diabetic ketoacidosis or lactic acidosis, certain toxins, or the acidosis of renal failure result in the production of unmeasured nonvolatile anions, which will cause an **increased** anion gap. Disorders such as renal tubular acidosis, which result in a loss of HCO$_3$, will display a **normal** anion gap.

C. **If an alkalosis exists, is it metabolic or respiratory?**

1. **PCO$_2$ < 35 mm Hg** reflects a respiratory alkalosis, usually due to hyperventilation. Common etiologies include anxiety, acidemia (compensation), CNS injury, pneumothorax, fever, pulmonary embolism, pregnancy, hepatic cirrhosis, and toxins. Overzealous mechanical ventilation is also a common cause of respiratory alkalosis.

2. **[HCO$_3$] > 26 mEq/L** indicates a metabolic alkalosis, usually of **iatrogenic** origin: diuretic or HCO$_3$ treatment, steroids, nasogastric suctioning, or severe vomiting are common etiologies. Less common causes include Cushing's disease, hypoparathyroidism, and aldosteronism.

   The analysis of metabolic alkaloses rests on whether or not the underlying disorder involves a volume-depleted, hypochloremic state (i.e., **chloride-responsive** etiologies such as those associated with vomiting and diuretics) or is secondary to decreased chloride resorption (i.e., **chloride-resistant** etiologies such as Cushing's syndrome, hypoparathyroidism, and severe potassium depletion). The former are far more common.

D. **Compensated acid-base disorders.** Except in the acute setting, most acid-base disorders that you encounter will be compensated to some degree; if the PCO$_2$ is increased due to a **respiratory acidosis** the kidney will attempt to excrete protons and increase [HCO$_3$] to bring the pH back toward normal. Similarly, if the [HCO$_3$] is decreased by a **metabolic acidosis,** the lungs will respond by blowing off CO_2 and lowering the pH. In both of these cases, the pH will be returned to near normal, although it will usually not be completely corrected. Thus, the patient with a pH of 7.37, a serum [HCO$_3$] of 30 mEq/L and a PCO$_2$ of 52 mm Hg is demonstrating a **compensated respiratory acidosis;** the PCO$_2$ is clearly abnormal (demonstrating a respiratory acidotic problem) while the mildly elevated [HCO$_3$] represents the body's attempt to restore a normal pH through a metabolic adjustment.

   Table 9-1 outlines the types and magnitudes of the compensating mechanisms in acid-base disorders.

E. **Mixed acid-base disorders.** Consider this example of a patient who has just suffered an acute myocardial infarction and has gone into respiratory arrest. His tissues are not being perfused, so he will quickly develop a metabolic acidosis due to the buildup of lactic acid. Because his lungs are not functioning either, he will also retain CO_2, resulting in a respiratory acidosis as well. His picture is thus a

Table 9-1. Acid-base disorder compensation

A. Alkalosis

1. Metabolic alkalosis. PCO_2 ↑ 0.25–1.0 mm Hg for each 1.0 mmol/L ↑ in $[HCO_3]$.

2. Acute respiratory alkalosis. $[HCO_3]$ ↓ by 2.0–4.0 mmol/L for each 10 mm Hg ↓ in PCO_2.

3. Chronic respiratory alkalosis. $[HCO_3]$ ↓ by 2.0–5.0 mmol/L for each 10 mm Hg ↓ in PCO_2.

B. Acidosis

1. Metabolic acidosis. PCO_2 ↓ 1.0–1.5 mm Hg for every 1.0 mmol/L ↓ in $[HCO_3]$.

2. Acute respiratory acidosis. $[HCO_3]$ ↑ by 1.0 mmol/L for each 10 mm Hg ↑ in PCO_2.

3. Chronic respiratory acidosis. $[HCO_3]$ ↑ by 4 mmol/L for each 10 mm Hg ↑ PCO_2.

mixed metabolic and respiratory acidosis, and his pH may be extraordinarily low, requiring immediate HCO_3 treatment and mechanical ventilation.

In a similar way, a patient may have a compensating acid-base disorder, such as a respiratory acidosis (increased PCO_2) combined with the metabolic alkalosis (increased $[HCO_3]$), as in an emphysema patient being treated for CHF with high-dose diuretics. In this case, the pH may be within the normal range.

Schrier [28] provides a good treatment of acid-base disorders and their clinical management.

| B | **Practical Points Concerning the Arterial Blood Gas Determination** |

I. Performing the arterial blood gas determination

A. The **Allen test** is a useful procedure for evaluating the collateral circulation in patients in whom arterial puncture might result in severe hypoperfusion of the hand if the collateral circulation were inadequate. It is conducted as follows (*Dorland's Illustrated Medical Dictionary,* App. C, **I.**):

> The pt. makes a tight fist so as to express the blood from the skin of the palm and fingers; the examiner exerts digital compression on either the radial or ulnar artery. If on opening the hand, the blood fails to return to the palm and fingers, there is indicated obstruction to the blood flow in the artery that has not been compressed.

The key to the test is the return (or failure of return) of the pink hue of a well-perfused palm.

B. The usual order of preference for **ABG puncture site** is radial artery, then brachial artery, and finally femoral artery. You should familiarize yourself with the exact location of these arteries and practice palpating them on yourself. Learn to feel for these arteries in a way that lets you "see" their course underneath your fingertips.

C. Take opportunities to practice your **arterial puncture technique** in non-emergency situations so that you will be able to act quickly and competently when speed is necessary. Being able to obtain a sample of arterial blood without unduly traumatizing your patient is a small but important clinical skill.

II. Interpreting arterial blood gas results

A. Recall that **the oxygen saturation curve for hemoglobin is a steep sigmoid** that starts to level off near a PO_2 of 70 mm Hg. This means that a patient may have a PO_2 of 65 mm Hg and still have greater than 90% O_2 saturation. Conversely, the difference between a PO_2 of 50 and PO_2 of 60 mm Hg is very clinically significant because it lies on the steep slope of the curve.

B. Always **note whether an ABG was drawn while the patient was receiving oxygen therapy.** This fact is often forgotten in the heat of the moment and obviously affects the PO_2 and oxygen saturation.

C. Always **analyze the ABG results together with the serum electrolytes and the anion gap.** If the patient is acidotic, the anion gap becomes the next step in constructing the differential diagnosis.

D. In analyzing the clinical status of a patient who has undergone an ABG, you must **know what baseline values are normal for your patient.** Many patients with chronic pulmonary disease exist quite happily with a PO_2 of 60 mm Hg, and it would be futile and often dangerous to attempt to improve their respiratory status much beyond this level.

The Medical Write-Up and Progress Notes

A

Annotated Outline and Example of the Medical Write-Up and Progress Notes

I. General points concerning the medical write-up

A. **Purpose.** The write-up has 3 major purposes.

1. **To convey information** to others, especially to **consultants**, who are not as familiar with the case as the responsible house officer, and to **covering house officers**, who may be asked to make a decision in the middle of the night concerning a patient with whom they are not familiar.

2. **To document and clarify the impression and approaches** of the medical team for future medical reference and medicolegal inquiries.

3. To force the writer **to quantify and organize** his or her own impressions in order to gain a better understanding of the case.

The student write-up, for better or worse, has an additional purpose: to show the student's preceptors how thoroughly the student has investigated and analyzed the case and how familiar he or she is with the differential diagnoses and the various management options that exist.

B. **Format.** Two major formats are currently in use for teaching hospital write-ups. The first, sometimes called the **traditional write-up,** is by far the most widely used. Its outline is shown in the sample write-up following Part A of this chapter. Its major advantage is that it is issue-oriented: within a general framework, its complexity expands and contracts in relation to the complexity of the medical case. Its major disadvantage is that information may be recorded and organized

Life and death crises actually occupy a reasonably small portion of clinical medicine, and an even smaller portion of the patient's concern over the quality of life. We must recognize that when a patient feels a problem is an emergency, it *is,* by definition, an emergency to the patient, whether or not the physician views the problem as life threatening. Even the highest quality of scientific medical management will not satisfy the patient unless these underlying concerns are answered.
Harley A. Haynes, M.D.

Perhaps the most difficult thing for medical students and house staff to learn and a lesson the experienced physician frequently relearns, often with discomfort but rarely with surprise, is that for everything we do, based upon sound rationales, for or to acutely ill patients, there are often equally persuasive competing rationales as to why we should *not* choose a certain treatment or intervention. Recognizing and dealing with those opposing issues constitutes a most challenging basis for developing clinical judgment. That developmental process begins with awareness of the issues and plans to detect and evaluate adverse effects at the earliest reasonable moment.
Roland H. Ingram, Jr., M.D.

in a rather haphazard way. Information pertaining to multiple separate medical problems, for instance, may be grouped in a single long paragraph, making future chart review more difficult.

The second write-up format, often called the **problem-oriented medical record (POMR)**, was developed by Dr. Larry Weed in order to standardize the collection and analysis of medical data and to aid in the development of a dynamic, readily accessible file of information on each significant medical problem affecting the patient. Its chief advantage is its comprehensiveness and the ease with which the current status of any medical problem can be assessed. Its chief disadvantage is that it is somewhat more cumbersome and difficult to use than the traditional format. A complete description of the problem-oriented system is beyond the scope of this chapter, but essentially it involves the recording of all medical data as entries under the headings of specific medical problems.

Although the problem-oriented system may be used with increasing frequency as medical records become computerized, its use at present is still the exception rather than the rule. Many physicians, however, are starting to incorporate certain elements of the POMR into a traditional write-up framework (e.g., an "active problem list" is now a standard part of many hospital charts), and hybrids of the two systems are now common. Students beginning their clinical rotations should check with their preceptors to determine which specific write-up format is preferred within their hospital system.

C. **Stance.** The good write-up is not simply an organized rehash of the information collected in the process of the work-up. Rather, it is a structured narrative in which the writer walks the delicate line between objective recording and subjective interpreting. From its very beginning, the good write-up takes a stance, organizing the details of the case into a coherent whole that implicitly or explicitly reflects the writer's impression of which issues are central and which are more peripheral. It is the ability to filter the data as it is being collected that allows the experienced clinician to write short but complete chart notes that command respect. While the second- or third-year student is usually not permitted the privilege of brevity, he or she should realize that even the most compulsively complete write-up can be organized in a way that persuades as well as informs. It should contain all the relevant data necessary for the reader to form an independent opinion concerning the case, but it should arrange the data in a way that lets the reader understand what has led the student to draw the conclusions that are offered. A common pitfall of student write-ups is an attempt to be overly "evenhanded"; to record objectively every bit of information obtained in the work-up, and to avoid deliberately taking any stance until the Assessment portion of the write-up. While this attempt at evenhandedness may seem admirable, it often results in a sort of laundry list of patient complaints and lab data that leaves the reader with little sense of the actual crucial issues. It is always appropriate to consider multiple diagnostic possibilities, but in relatively clear-cut cases the student should concentrate on those issues that will make the diagnosis and not be distracted by complaints that clearly seem unrelated or peripheral. Although the student may be expected to produce a long differential diagnosis list in the Assessment section, the entire write-up should be geared toward differentiating between the two or three most likely possibilities.

II. Progress notes

A. **Purpose.** Once the initial admission write-up is completed, the student or house officer is expected to write a brief progress note every day. As the name implies, these notes summarize what progress has been made in the case since the last note. The central issues of the progress note address the following questions:

1. What are the patient's current symptoms and complaints? Are there any changes?

2. Is there any change in the physical exam?

3. Are there any new lab data?

4. Is there any change in the formulation of the case or the relationship of the patient's various medical problems to one another?

5. What are the current diagnostic and therapeutic plans for the patient?

B. Format. As in the case of the initial admission write-up, there are two main formats for progress notes: the **traditional format**, which is simply a set of paragraphs summarizing the progress, and the **problem-oriented format**, in which entries for each medical problem are divided into four sections:

1. Subjective data, i.e., the patient's impressions of current symptoms.

2. Objective data, i.e., the clinical exam and lab data.

3. Assessment, i.e., the writer's impression of the data and their relation to the case.

4. Plan, both diagnostic and therapeutic.

A progress note with information arranged in the order **S**ubjective–**O**bjective–**A**ssessment–**P**lan is often referred to as a **SOAP note.** No matter whether the initial write-up follows the traditional or the problem-oriented format, many clinicians believe that all progress notes should be written in some variant of the SOAP note format because it makes chart review much easier.

C. Off-service notes. The off-service note is a specialized version of the progress note. Above all, it should be **brief,** usually one page or less in length, and contain:

1. A short summary of the patient's case, usually one paragraph.

2. A short summary of the hospital course, again usually one paragraph.

3. A problem list that details ongoing, active problems and any outstanding diagnostic tests or work-up.

4. A list of current medications and dosages.

Remember that the purpose of the off-service note is to allow the physician who is coming on-service to orient himself to the patient's case in an expeditious way.

III. Sample write-up and progress notes. Reproduced on pp. 134–151 is a good second-year student's admission write-up, together with two progress notes from the same case. Note that the write-up, while primarily organized in the traditional format, contains elements of the problem-oriented system. The chief complaint and the present illness essentially become problem no. 1 on the patient's problem list, while the past medical history comprises the rest of the patient's active medical problems. Part B of this chapter is keyed to the following sample write-up and contains specific practical points about the format and content of each section of the write-up. As is usually the case with medical notes, many abbreviations and acronyms are used. The glossary on the inside cover lists most of these standard terms.

While the admission note below represents a better than average second-year write-up, it would be considered inappropriately wordy and compulsively thorough by third- or fourth-year standards. In particular, note that the review of systems (ROS) is written out in its entirety. While most second-year students are required to describe the complete ROS, the third-year student is generally permitted to record a shorter list of pertinent positives and negatives, while the fourth-year student may simply record the essential ones and note that the "remainder of the ROS was negative in detail." Also note that the Assessment and Plan section ("Impression") is too brief and could be fleshed out. Compare it to the progress note that follows.

The first progress note reproduced after the sample write-up is organized in the traditional style (p. 148), while the second is written as a SOAP note (p. 150). In a complicated case with many consultants writing notes it is not unusual to see multiple styles being used on the same case, and a student should get comfortable with all of them. Note that whether or not a formal SOAP note is written, all notes organize information in the order "**s**ubjective, **o**bjective, **a**ssessment, and **p**lan," and that the acronym is useful regardless of the style used.

PROGRESS NOTES

INPATIENT

— Medical Student Admission Note —
3/3/87

Source: pt, who seems reliable, and old chart.

This is the second admission for Mrs. Elsa
Jones, a 55 y.o. black seamstress who enters with
C.C: "weakness," "cough," and "feverish feeling" of
several days duration.

H.P.I: Mrs. Jones was in her usual state of
health until this past Friday (2/28/87)
when she noted fatigue during her work-
day and in the evening, without other
associated symptoms. The following morning
this tired feeling persisted and the pt.
Confined herself to her home "to rest" for
the majority of Saturday. She slept
well Saturday night but awoke with
nasal stuffiness and an occasional
cough productive of clear mucoid
Sputum. As the day progressed nausea
accompanied by 3-4 episodes of vomiting
occured, as did several mild chills without
overt shaking. The pt. first recalls feeling
feverish at approximately this time, though
she did not take her own temperature.

PROGRESS NOTES

INPATIENT

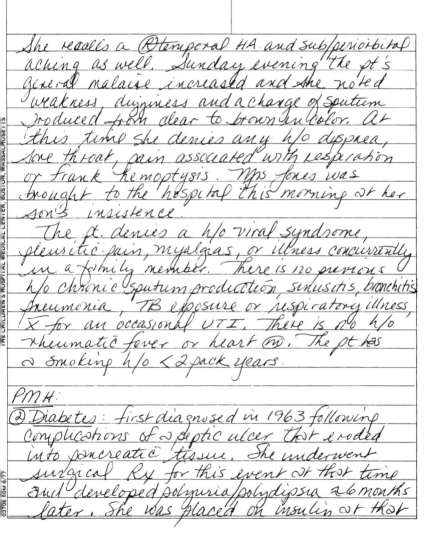

She recalls a (R) temporal HA and sub/periorbital aching as well. Sunday evening the pt's general malaise increased and she noted weakness, dizziness and a change of sputum produced from clear to brown in color. At this time she denies any h/o dyspnea, sore throat, pain associated with respiration or frank hemoptysis. Mrs. Jones was brought to the hospital this morning at her son's insistence.

The pt. denies a h/o viral syndrome, pleuritic pain, myalgias, or illness concurrently in a family member. There is no previous h/o chronic sputum production, sinusitis, bronchitis, pneumonia, TB exposure or respiratory illness, X for an occasional UTI. There is no h/o rheumatic fever or heart (D). The pt has a smoking h/o < 2 pack years.

PMH:
② Diabetes: first diagnosed in 1963 following complications of a peptic ulcer that eroded into pancreatic tissue. She underwent surgical Rx for this event at that time and developed polyuria/polydipsia ≈6 months later. She was placed on insulin at that

PROGRESS NOTES

INPATIENT

time and currently is on 80u NPH, 15 CZI qd, which maintains her serumglucose/urine S+A's under good control.

③ HTN: dx'ed 7 yrs ago on clinic visit, well controlled (< 150/96) on 50mg Guanethidine qd from then until present.

④ Hyperlipoproteinemia: dx'ed in 1972 on routine lab studies. Noted to have chol 442 mg% TG 750 mg%; was re-evaluated the following year c̄ Chol 368, TG's 5,900 and dx'ed c̄ Type I hyperlipoproteinemia. Placed on Atromid-S subsequently c̄ reasonable control (TG of 411 mg% reported 9/79). Presently taking Atromid qid; without recent TG in chart.

⑤ R.A.: Mrs. Jones has a 30 yr h/o Rheumatoid arthritis, dx'ed at MGH clinic. History vague; symptomatic relief c̄ ASA since that time and pt reports not a problem currently (see ROS)

<u>Childhood illness(es)</u>: ⊅ significant. Pt. recalls a kidney infection ≈20 yrs ago but few other

PROGRESS NOTES

INPATIENT

details. No h/o freq., sore throats, TB, rheumatic fever.

Allergies. Sulfa drugs → diffuse rash

Previous Admissions:

admission	year	hospital
Pregnancy, hysterectomy	1961	MGH
ulcer complications, Pancreatectomy $\bar{c}$ 1963	1963	MGH
Dental Work	1977	PBBH

Other PMH: No h/o accidents/trauma or broken bones.

FHX

gassed, WWI (74) —— (56) Ht disease / Stroke

multiple (61) MI   (55)   (58) multiple MI repeated Kidney infections   (65) pneumonia x1

No family h/o AODM, Ca, TB; No h/o HTN, sickle cell disease

⊕ CAD, MI as noted in diagram

Social Hx:

Widow of 6 yrs, Mrs. Jones' husband died of an MI. Lives with her son, age 26. States

PROGRESS NOTES

INPATIENT

they are extremely close.
Has worked as a stitcher for 38 yrs at Sharon
Dress Co. in Roxbury. Pt makes her own hours
and enjoys her job a great deal. No h/o toxic
exposure or work.
Describes herself as generally happy/content
person.

Current meds: EtOH ⊖ Tobacco Hx: <2pk-yrs.
Insulin NPH 80u + CZI 15u SC qAM
Guanethidine 50 mg p̄o qd
Atromid S ī tab p̄o qd

ROS

constitutional: fatigue often; onset of present
fatigue notable. No recent wt change,
night sweats, chills, s̄ insomnia.
integument: ⊕ itching, nightly; localized to
back, of 1-yr. duration. ↑ thinning hair
x 3 yrs. s̄ rash (x̄ c̄ Sulfa drugs), sores,
bruising/bleeding.
Head: s̄ h/a x̄ c̄ present illness (see HPI). s̄
fainting, LOC; seizures or h/o trauma.
Eyes: glasses x 10-12 yrs. last eye exam 3 weeks
ago (frequent excessive tearing, s̄ apparent
agg/allev factors). Notes blurred vision often,

PROGRESS NOTES

INPATIENT

but improved since eye exam. Occasional ®side pain in region of ext. canthus - "like a knife going through my eye" - relieved by sleep.

Ears: hearing "pretty good." ⊖pain, discharge, vertigo.

Resp: see HPI

Breasts: no masses, pain, discharge. Does self-exam

CV: ⊕ ankle edema at end of day. No h/o palpitations, dyspnea, PND, chest pain or discomfort cyanosis, varicose veins. ⊕ DM, smoking presently; hyperlipoproteinemia as noted.

GI: dental plate, top teeth; partial on bottom. ⊕ vomiting c̄ present illness - clear, fluid, less than 3-4 tablespoons each time. No h/o heartburn, hematemesis, Abd pain/discomfort since ulcer difficulties in 1963, food intolerance, jaundice, hematochezia. No recent Δ in stool (normal frequency, color, consistency).

GU:
1. Urinary ⊕ nocturia, 2-3 x/night; has had nocturia "as long as I can remember." No h/o dysuria, pyuria, stones, flank pain, urgency/frequency.
2. Menstrual: menopause c̄ hysterectomy in 1961, accompanied by hot flushes, depression. Reports reason for hysterectomy was "tumor" discovered at time of son's birth. Last pap smear 3 months

PROGRESS NOTES

INPATIENT

ago (neg) No present c/o vag. discharge, itching.
Endocrine: hirsutism c̄ androgens p̄ hysterectomy.
No present problems c̄ polyuria, polydipsia.
_MS:_ ⊕ occasional calve "pulls" - Rx c̄ hot soaks.
⊕ arthritis c̄ "all joints," accompanied by
warmth, soreness, morning stiffness most
mornings, Rx c̄ Ben-Gay ®, hot soaks q AM,
ASA c̄ good relief.
neuro:
motor: s̄ atrophy, involuntary movements
sensory: ⊕ numbness in toes often. s̄ anesthesia/
hyperesthesia.
mental status: mentation s̄ Δ, memory,
writing intact.

Physical Exam:
Mrs Jones is a moderately obese middle-aged
black woman who is resting quietly in her
chair s̄ apparent distress. She holds a
tissue with several streaks of blood visible
in her hand.
_VS:_ Temp 102.8°   weight: 61.2 kg
     Pulse 94, regular, strong
     BP   122/72 ♀ ® arm
          110/70 o̶ ® arm
     Resp. 25, somewhat shallow

PROGRESS NOTES

INPATIENT

Integument: Skin warm, dry, s̄ bruises, rashes, cyanosis. Nails nl.

HEENT:

  Head: normocephalic, s̄ evidence of trauma or scalp lesions. Hair thin, oily.

  Eyes: Visual acuity c̄ glasses ∼20/40 each eye. Conjunctiva nl. PERRLA. Palpebral fissures ≈ equal. EOM's intact. ⊕ Fundus: clear, c̄ sharp disc, ⊖ hemorrhage or exudate. ⓡ Fundus: not visualized - ? cataract ⓡ eye.

  Ears: Hearing intact. Minimal ceramen, TM clear c̄ good light reflex.

  Nose: nares patent, septum midline, ⊖ sinus tenderness/discharge.

  mouth/throat: dental plate - upper teeth, lower molars. Tongue well papillated, moist. Uvula midline. Throat s̄ injection/exudate.

Lymphadenopathy: s̄ cervical, axillary or inguinal.

Neck: trachea midline; ⊕ slt ↑ in thyroid size (easily palpated); s̄ nodules/tenderness.

Back: Spine s̄ curvatures; ⊖ CVA tenderness.

Lungs: Chest symmetrical ↓ respiratory excursion evident, ⓡⓛ symmetry preserved. percussion: nl, s̄ dull areas. Diaphragm

PROGRESS NOTES

INPATIENT

descends 1-2 cm > on Ⓛ

auscultation: Ⓑ end inspiratory rales, Ⓡ axilla.

Ⓔ tactile fremitus, egophony, whispered

pectoriloquy.

<u>Breasts</u> pendulous, symmetric, s̄ masses,

discharge or tenderness.

<u>CV:</u> JVP 7-8 cm

PMI · not visible or palpable. s̄ lift or

impulse palpable.

S₁: nl intensity. S₂: nl intensity, nl split

c̄ inspiration. ⊕ Soft S₄ ⊖ S₃.

Grade 2/6 SEM at LLSB s̄ radiation to

axilla or neck.

pulses:

	Carotid		radial	femoral	popliteal	D.P.	P.T.
Ⓡ	2+, nl upstroke, s̄ bruits		2+	1+, s̄ bruits	1+	2+	s̄
Ⓛ	2+, nl upstroke, s̄ bruits		2+	1+, s̄ bruits	1+	2+	s̄

<u>Abdomen:</u>

s̄ liver, spleen edge

<u>obese, bowel sounds</u> ⊕

liver: 10-11 cm by

percussion

cecum

palpable

25-30 cm scar

c̄ keloid

(ulcer surgery)

10-15 cm scar

(hysterectomy)

PROGRESS NOTES

INPATIENT

Genital Exam:
 external: 5 discharge, lesions
 pelvic: deferred to private gynecologist. Last pap
  12/87, negative.
Rectal Exam: sphincter good tone. guaiac neg.
MS: nl. ROM all 4 extremities. Feet slt
 ↓ temperature; color nl; hair present on toes.
 ⊕ joint hypertrophy - DIP's ⊖ tenderness,
 ⊖ subcutaneous nodules. muscular strength
 4+/5+ all four limbs.
Neuro:
 Motor: (see MS) F → N√√, H → S√√. Rhomberg
  ⊖. Gait slow, slt shuffling
 Sensory: pinprick ↓ in both feet; nl position,
 vibration
 CN: II → XII √√
 Reflexes:

⊖ babinski as illustrated

Mental Status: oriented X3; serial 7's intact;
 pt is alert.

PROGRESS NOTES

INPATIENT

Laboratory data

CBC: HCT 35.7

WBC: 11.8 (79 polys, 6 Ba, 7 ly, 7mo, 1 baso)

PT: 11.3/12.5   PTT 25/25.3   ESR 24

U/A: straw/yellow ; SG 1.020 ; pH 6.0
      Prot 3+ Heme 1+   0-1 RBC/HPF
      Gm ⊖ Rods in unspun specimen
      analysis ;   3-5 WBC/HPF
      S/A - 1+/⊖

Serum Chems: $\dfrac{142 | 102}{3.7 | 29}{<}^{12}_{187}$ ⟨ $^{12}_{187}$ Ca/PO₄ 9.6/3.8
      $\dfrac{142|102}{3.7|29}$ ⟨ $^{12}_{187}$ ⟨ $^{1.0}$ Cholesterol 210
                    UA 6.8
                TG's - not checked

EKG: Axis - 20° .14/.08/.90 ? LVH ($V_1 + V_5 = 36$mm)
      Rate 120, NSR   insignificant Q in II, F
      Remainder $\bar{s}$ abnormality

CXR: ⊕ RLL superior segment alveolar
      infiltrate.   Borderline cardiomegaly.
      ⊖ effusions

Sputum gm stain : 4+ polys, numerous gm⊕
                   diplococci

urine, sputum cultures : pending.

Assessment/Plan

Summary: This 55 yo. black ♀ presents c̄
fever, productive cough and progressive

PROGRESS NOTES

INPATIENT

malaise of 3-4 days duration.

① Productive cough: Recent onset of cough, productive of sputum which changed from mucoid → brown, fever, nausea, vomiting are all c/w dx of pneumonia. PE data includes presence of ⓡ axillary rales but no signs suggestive of consolidation. There was no evidence from Hx or PE supporting obstruction (acute or insidious) → no wt. Δ, h/o aspiration, other evidence of cachexia; also no wheezing or rhonchi on lung exam. There was no evidence for non-pulmonary etiology (mitral stenosis, e.g.) Lab data increases the likelihood that this is a bacterial pneumonia: sputum c̄ 4+ polys and gm ⊕ diplococci; CXR c̄ ⓡLL infiltrate.

　　Important to R/o obstruction, and TB as other common possibilities. Pul. embolism uncommon infectious cause are less likely.

Plan: ① Place TB test c̄ mumps/candida control
　　　② Begin antibiotics with Ampicillin 500mg q6h IV (see below for discussion of antibiotic choice)

PROGRESS NOTES

INPATIENT

③ blood cultures x 2

② <u>Asymptomatic Bacteriuria</u> – discovered during laboratory work-up. Though pt's symptoms will choose antibiotics for presumptive pneumonia that covers typical gm ⊖ rods causing UTI (generally enteric organisms). Note that pt. is predisposed to UTI's if her diabetes is not well controlled (see below).

Plan : ① send urine for definitive culture / sensitivities
② begin Ampicillin 500 mg Q6h IV
③ check urine S+A's

③ Opacity, ® eye: pt c̄ numerous visual complaints but s̄ marked loss of ® eye vision; also last eye exam 3 weeks ago. However, c̄ hx/of diabetes, ↑ incidence of cataract. Will therefore:

Plan : ① attempt to contact ophthalmologist
② in-house ophthalmology consult

④ <u>AODM</u>. Will assess degree of control while pt. in hospital. Note that infection likely to increase insulin requirement and thus may show some ↑ in BS (may account for asymptomatic bacteriuria noted above).

PROGRESS NOTES

INPATIENT

Plan: ① urine S+A's
    ② √ FBS
    ③ 1800 cal/day diet (ADA)

⑤ Type I Hyperlipoproteinemia: Last triglyceride recorded in chart was 9/84
Plan: ① Check TG level
    ② Continue Atromid-S

⑥ Hypertension: Under good control with BP 122/72 sitting; 110/70 supine. Ophthalmology consult planned (see ③ above)

⑦ Rheumatoid arthritis: though pt says currently not a problem, she also states arthritis is present in "all" joints, accompanied by warmth, soreness; also morning stiffness most mornings. Rx c̄ ASA at present. Will
    Plan: ① Rheumatology consult to evaluate Rx.

Overall Impression: A 55 year old woman with pneumococcal pneumonia and possible UTI.

        John Smith
        2nd Year Medical Student

PROGRESS NOTES

INPATIENT

3/4/87 Medical Student Progress Note

Hx. No real change in Sx. Still c̄ cough and fever. Still bringing up small amounts of brown sputum.

PE: T 101° P 90, regular BP 120/70 ℞ and o—
    RR: 24 WEIGHT: 61.9 Kg (↓0.2 Kg)
    Exam. s̄ change. Still c̄ Expiratory
        rales ℞ >Ⓛ
    T.B. Test PPD ⊖ at 24 hrs.
        Candida control ⊕

Lab. CBC   34.2
        15.7 ╱──── Diff (61 p 25 B 8 L 5 m 1 Eo)
            ╱ 187 K

    U/A S.g. 1.015   pH 6.0
        2+ protein 1+ heme 1+ sugar -acetone
        0-1 RBC / 2-5 WBC per HPF
        few gram ⊖ rods per HPF in unspun
                specimen

    Chemistry 140 | 100 ⟨ 15
            3.8 | 26 ⟨ 205
                    1.1
        triglyceride: pending
    Sputum Gram Stain 4+ polys, gram ⊕ diplococci
    Sputum Cultures ⊕ Pneumococcus sensitive to
                    Ampicillin
    Urine cultures: pending

PROGRESS NOTES

INPATIENT

Impression: ① Pneumococcal Pneumonia : Temp
now ↓ but WBC ↑ ; will continue
Ampicillin 500 mg IV q6h. CBC and
CXR tomorrow.
                ② UTI : No Sx ; cultures pending
                        James Smith
                        Medical Student II

PROGRESS NOTES

INPATIENT

3/5/87   Medical Student Progress Note

VS: Temp 99.2 P 85, regular BP 120/70 ᴱ and Ō

RR 20   Weight 62.0 Kg

Problem #1: Pneumococcal Pneumonia:

   S: Feels better. No more cough, very little sputum.

   O: Exam: still c̄ scattered expiratory wheezes.

     TB Test PPD ⊖ at 48 hours.

     CBC $\overline{34.8}$
          $12.1/221K$ diff (68p 18B 9L 5M)

     Sputum Gram Stain: 2+ polys; + diplococci

     CXR: Still c̄ RLL infiltrate.

   A: Symptomatically improved, Temp and WBC ↓

   P: Continue Ampicillin

Problem #2: UTI

   S: Still s̄ Sx

   O: urine culture from 3/3/87:

     >10⁵ Klebsiella sensitive to ampicillin

     U/A: 3 change from 3/4/87; still

     c̄ gram ⊖ rods in unspun; 2+polys

   A: Klebsiella UTI sensitive to current antibiotics

   P: Continue Ampicillin; repeat urine cultures tomorrow.

Problem #3 AODM:

   S: No new Sx or c/o

   O: urine S+A: 1+/⊖

PROGRESS NOTES

INPATIENT

Blood sugar 172 this AM
A and P : Well controlled.
Other Problems s̄ change.

— James Smith
  Medical Student II

B   **Practical Points Concerning
                                       the Medical Write-Up and
                                       Progress Notes**

I. Introductory information and chief complaint

A. All chart notes should be written on **hospital progress note paper** that has been marked or stamped with the patient's name and hospital number. You may find it useful to prepare a supply of this stamped paper when you are first assigned a patient and to carry it around on your clipboard so that you can work on notes when you are away from the chart. Of course, all entries should be dated and signed.

B. It is customary to **title each note** with the level of seniority of *the writer* (e.g., "Medical Student Admission Note" or "Heme Attending Note"). Consultants who review the chart can thus key in on critical entries.

C. **Record your source** if you derive any of the information in your note from a source other than the patient or the old chart. Although a reliability caveat may be appropriate here (e.g., "patient appeared confused and vague"), it should never be humorous or flip.

D. The introductory sentence and chief complaint (given with its duration) should provide a **10-second sketch of the patient** and the patient's reason for seeking medical help. A word or two about the patient's past medical history may be appropriate here as well (e.g., "a 55 y.o. black seamstress with a long history of hypertension"). You will often use this introductory sentence to allude to the patient in discussions with those not familiar with the case.

II. History of the present illness

A. **Chronologic organization** is the key to a well-written history of the present illness (HPI). Begin with a sentence describing the onset of the constellation of symptoms that you perceive as the present illness. If the present illness is simply the latest episode in a long-standing medical problem, begin with a sentence about how long the patient has suffered from the disease (e.g., "The patient has a 20-year history of asthma usually involving 1 or 2 attacks each spring."). Then organize the salient features of the case, always noting the dates on which the features appeared. For a long-standing problem, this will mean a careful chart review with dates of hospitalizations, surgical procedures, therapies, and definitive diagnostic tests all highlighted. The goal here is to give the reader a feeling for the tempo of the disease process.

B. **All pertinent positives** and **some pertinent negatives** from the ROS of the organ system(s) involved in the present illness belong in the HPI. Often it is not clear whether a certain pertinent negative is really important enough to note in the HPI. In these cases a good rule of thumb is to ask yourself whether the information in question helps exclude a possible diagnosis that has entered your

---

The diagnosis is nearly always contained in the patients' words and physical findings. The physician must translate their words and the data obtained with the eyes, ears, and hands into a language that describes disorders of organ functions. Remember: the hand of disease can be quicker than the eye of the physician.

Kenneth H. Falchuk, M.D.

Among the various diagnostic possibilities pertaining to any seriously ill patient, the curable ones ought to be pursued first and most vigorously, whatever the diagnostic probabilities.

Alexander S. Nadas, M.D.

mind while considering the patient's symptoms. If it does, then the information belongs in the HPI.

III. Past medical history

A. All **active** and **significant inactive medical problems** should be listed in the past medical history (PMH). This section can be anywhere from a few sentences to a few pages in length, depending on the severity and the significance of the problems. For each problem, the significant issues that you should concentrate on include:

    1. The date on which the problem was diagnosed.

    2. The results of definitive tests that will indicate to the reader the severity of the problem (e.g., "cardiac cath in 1979 showed a 38% ejection fraction").

    3. The dates of any surgeries or hospitalizations.

    4. Current treatment regimens.

    5. An assessment of the problem's significance at present, and its potential for interacting with the present illness.

B. Other parts of the medical history included in the PMH include:

    1. A list of significant **childhood illnesses**.

    2. **Allergies** and the nature of the allergic reaction.

    3. A list of **past hospitalizations** and **surgical procedures** (even if mentioned elsewhere).

IV. Family history

A. The family history (FHx) is usually presented in a standard **pedigree format**:

    (30) = female, 30 years old
    MI ⊠ = male, died at age 42 of myocardial infarct
    → (55) = patient, female, 55 years old

For most cases, you will want to list the patient, the patient's siblings, and the patient's parents and children.

B. Any family history of **diabetes, cancer, cardiovascular problems,** or other disease with significant genetic penetration should also be listed in the FHx. A family history of the disease (or symptoms) that the patient has presented with should always be sought.

V. Social history. The social history (SHx) should be very brief unless a lengthy treatment would be of crucial importance to the case. Its goal is to give the reader an idea of the patient as a person. For most patients this section of the write-up will involve a few words about the patient's **living situation** and **work.** Names and telephone numbers of close family members can also be listed here. Recall from Chap. 1 (Part A, **VI. C**) instances in which this section assumes a larger role, such as occupational exposures and pulmonary disease.

VI. Current medications and habits. The medication list should document all significant pharmacologically active substances used by the patient. These include all medicines, vitamins, skin creams, laxatives, sleeping medications, contraceptives, and recreational drugs, including ethanol and tobacco. Each of these substances should be listed with the dosage and route of administration. It is customary to use the Latin acronyms for dosage frequency, e.g., "bid" (*bis in die*) for "2 times per day" (see glossary). The smoking history should be listed in pack-years. Drinking history may be quantitated in familiar units (six-packs, quarts).

VII. Review of systems. The review of systems should be **listed by organ system.** Once again, this list will be long or short depending on the complexity of the case and the level of the writer. Experienced clinicians may simply write "ROS negative." When first beginning your clinical training, at a minimum, you should list all the ROS positives and enough of the pertinent negatives to show the reader that you did a complete ROS and that all the important facets of the case are listed. List the ROS telegraphically. For example:

GI: ⊖ Nausea, vomiting, diarrhea, constipation, abd. pain
⊕ Tarry stools several times in last week

VIII. Physical examination

A. Introductory information and vital signs. Begin with a statement describing the overall appearance of the patient. The vital signs (including orthostatic changes in blood pressure and pulse) should be listed before the rest of the exam. For most patients with cardiovascular or renal problems, the admission weight should be listed with the vital signs.

B. Organ system examination. Starting with a description of the integument and then proceeding in a generally head-to-toe direction (leaving the neurologic exam results for last), transcribe the results of your physical exam. Just as in the ROS, the second-year student should include all significant positive and negative findings while the more advanced student can concentrate on the major positive findings, listing only the most fundamental pertinent negatives.

C. One key to a good physical exam write-up is **specificity.** Always quantitate and localize (e.g., "a 6 × 6-cm round erythematous patch on the left buttock"). Draw **diagrams** wherever they are helpful. Specifically, the dermatologic exam, breast exam, abdominal exam, and neurologic exam are often illustrated with diagrams and stick figures to indicate the exact location of the findings.

IX. Laboratory data (see also Chapters 4–9)

A. Hematologic studies are usually listed together in shorthand form as follows:

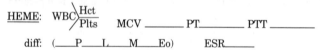

Any special hematologic tests or comments on the blood smear, which should be examined whenever the differential is abnormal or suggestive, are recorded below these results.

B. Urinalysis (U/A) data are recorded in tabular form:

<u>U/A</u>: color and appearance; specific gravity; pH and dipstick results; sediment analysis; quantitation (number of cells or structures per high power field)

The time and conditions of collection (e.g., catheter or clean-voided specimen) and total urine volume in a specified time period may also be recorded here. If you do one urinalysis and the lab does another, include both sets of data, noting the source of each.

C. Serum chemistry data can be divided into:

1. Seven "core" tests, which are conveniently recorded in a lattice as follows:

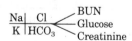

2. The remainder of the serum chemistry results, which are recorded underneath and beside this lattice. Often these other tests are best grouped by organ system (e.g., the liver function tests). You should circle lab values that are abnormal or significant to the diagnosis in question.

D. Electrocardiographic data should be recorded in the following sequence:

1. Rate and rhythm.

2. Axis.

3. P-Q, QRS, and Q-T intervals.

4. Comments concerning the following areas:

   a. Q waves and S-T segment morphology.

   b. R wave progression.

   c. QRS morphology and conduction blocks.

   d. Evidence for hypertrophy.

   e. Evidence for drug effects.

   f. Other significant findings.

5. Overall impression, *including degree of change from the last recorded ECG.*

E. Chest x-ray results are recorded either verbally or by means of a labeled diagram. Always include a statement concerning the degree of change from the last chest film.

F. In a similar telegraphic fashion, record the remainder of the lab data including:

1. **Arterial blood gas determinations** (record the FiO_2 together with the results and the time the sample was drawn).

2. **Microbiologic data** (include antibiotic sensitivities if known).

3. **Pathology reports.**

4. **Other radiologic tests.**

5. **Other special diagnostic tests.**

X. Assessment and plan. Up until this point in the write-up, the **analytic** portion of the work-up has been collected and organized. Now the history, physical exam, and lab data are considered together in the **synthetic** portion of the work-up, in which each problem is systematically assessed and a management plan for each is formulated. This section of the write-up may be considered in four parts: (a) a **summary** is written; (b) a complete **problem list** is generated; (c) an **assessment** is made of each problem on the list; and (d) a **plan,** both for further diagnosis and for therapy, is formulated.

A. Summary. Write a **brief, two- to three-line** summary after the last piece of lab data is recorded and before the assessment and plan are made for each problem. Summarizing serves to refocus both your own and the reader's attention to the case at hand, emphasizing the central concern(s) of the HPI. An example is illustrated in the sample write-up.

B. Problem list. You will be familiar with the concept of a problem list from earlier medical studies, but several specific points are useful to remember here:

1. A problem list is the **collected set of findings** that you believe need to be addressed as part of a patient's overall case. **Problems are derived from four general areas: the history, the physical exam, laboratory findings, and a synthesis of any or all of these three.** Thus findings such as chest pain, a supraclavicular node, and a low serum sodium value are all possible entries, as in pneumonia, a diagnosis arrived at from synthesizing data from the history, physical exam, and laboratory. As you gain experience, it will become clear that certain entries previously considered distinct from one another in fact may be subsumed under one new heading on your problem list. What is important at the outset is identifying all abnormalities or problems by methodically examining the data available. The problem list should serve as an **overall outline** for thinking about the case; thus it will ideally consist of a collection of the fewest number of entries that together explain all your findings.

2. The construction of a problem list is not simply an academic exercise; it is the

initial step in management of the patient. Therefore, if there is a problem that you have no intention of addressing (e.g., poor dentition), it probably does not belong on your problem list.

3. The problem that is central to the present illness usually occupies the number 1 spot on the problem list. Related and distinct problems from the history, physical exam, and laboratory data are then **ranked** in order of the importance you ascribe to them.

C. **Assessment.** Now that the problem list exists, the task remaining is to address each problem in turn, considering its significance and reflecting on diagnostic possibilities if the etiology is unclear. This analysis of each problem is at least partially put to paper in the form of the assessment. As is illustrated in the sample write-up, each problem is discussed in turn, and from this "thinking on paper" arises the logical sequence of further diagnostic steps and therapeutic interventions that are listed below each problem as the **plan.**

The assessment is usually written in the form of one paragraph for each problem.

1. Begin by stating the **diagnoses** that seem to be the most probable explanation for the problem in question (unless, of course, your heading is a diagnosis, such as "pneumonia").

2. Methodically mention the compelling **history, physical exam,** and **laboratory findings** that are related to the problem in question and that help support the conclusion you are drawing about the significance of a given problem.

3. Mention **other diagnostic possibilities** that you have entertained, and, again using data from the history, physical exam, and laboratory, state why they are unlikely or not yet excluded.

4. By this point the **further diagnostic studies** necessary to arrive at a decisive diagnosis will be fairly clear. These studies for the entries form the first part of your plan list.

5. Lastly, consider conditions related to the problem in question that may be important to explore. This part of the assessment requires experience and a firm knowledge of pathophysiology and clinical presentations of disease. For example, if a patient's pneumococcal pneumonia was his third such event in the past 18 months, it might be worthwhile to rule out the possibility of an underlying multiple myeloma (which predisposes to recurrent pneumonia especially with encapsulated bacteria) by ordering a serum immunoelectrophoresis.

D. The **plan** logically proceeds from the reasoning presented in the paragraph following each problem on the problem list; it is simply a checklist of things to be done. The first entries are further **diagnostic** steps, as mentioned above (**C.4**). Following these are the **therapeutic interventions** on which you and your team have decided.

To summarize and elaborate on the areas that the assessment and plan address, we have listed below topics to consider when formulating these sections:

1. **Definitive diagnoses.** For problems that are unsolved, try to narrow the diagnostic possibilities and decide what needs to be done to arrive at a final diagnosis. Consider the need for subspecialty consultations here.

2. **Correction or compensation of pathophysiology.** This subject is the cornerstone of medical management. Thinking about pathophysiology, try to understand what perturbation has caused the problem in question and what might be done to compensate for or correct that causative factor.

3. **Therapeutic measures.** In addition to **2** above, consider the following areas with respect to therapy:

   a. Pain relief.

   b. Specific medications useful for the problem in question.

   c. Ancillary help (e.g., physical or occupational therapist, nutritionist).

   d. Prevention of complications (e.g., bedsore prophylaxis for those who must be on their back constantly).

   e. Long-term care (e.g., potential need for outpatient assistance, nursing home, VNA).

   As is evident from the sample write-up, each problem is addressed in turn, and a list of further steps is created.

E. Conclusion. As you come to the end of the assessment and plan, having addressed each problem, two measures are useful to help conclude your write-up. First, conclude with a brief impression of the case, as explained below (**XI**). Second, and perhaps more important, define for yourself the **endpoint** for your patient's present hospitalization. Although you may revise the endpoint deliberately, if it is not considered from the day of admission, you will find that the reasons for the patient's hospitalization seem to shift and change emphasis, causing the process of concluding the hospitalization to become very frustrating.

XI. Concluding information. In a complicated case it is sometimes useful to conclude the write-up with a few sentences of an **"overall impression,"** in which the case priorities and the long-term goals and sequence of therapies that you suggest implementing are briefly mentioned. This is a chance to integrate the patient's medical problems into a unified picture of the patient as a person rather than simply as a set of organ systems.

XII. Progress notes

   A. Keep your progress notes **brief** and **telegraphic**. Concentrate on any new data that you have, and any change in clinical symptoms or signs. Even if the patient's chart has a separate lab result section in which the lab tests are routinely recorded, you should still summarize new results in your progress notes. If a test has been done but the results are not available, note that the test is "pending." No matter what format is used, a good progress note should enable the reader to skim the day's data in a minute or two and answer the following questions:

   1. Is there any **new diagnostic information**?

   2. Is the patient getting **better or worse**?

   3. Are the **chosen therapies** working?

   4. What **further diagnostic and therapeutic steps** are in progress or planned?

   B. Flow charts are extremely useful, especially for patients with multiple interrelated medical problems. For instance, a patient with severe renal failure might benefit from a flow chart that allows quick day-by-day comparisons of those clinical parameters affected by renal failure. Such a flow chart might be set up as follows:

DATE	7/1	7/2	7/3	7/4
Electrolytes	$\dfrac{138}{5.6} \bigg| \dfrac{94}{25}$			
BUN/Creatine	56/3.8			
CBC	32.5 12.1 ∕ 242k			
ABGs	8:20 A.M. $PO_2 = 86$ 40% FiO_2 $PCO_2 = 28$ pH = 7.31			

   Although this sort of chart does not take the place of daily notes, it can be an invaluable aid to consultants who see the patient only every few days and to you and your intern when you wish to summarize the case.

In this chapter, Part A outlines the two types of presentations: the **brief presentation** on work rounds and the more **formal presentation** delivered to the attending physician. Part B provides a description of the teaching points emphasized during attending rounds and some of the general areas that need to be addressed when presenting.

Although practical information and hints have usually been confined to Part B in Chaps. 1–10, some can be found in part A of this chapter as well. In fact, presenting a case is an art, and as such it can be described only partially and learned only with practice.

A   **Annotated Outline of Medical Case Presentations**

I. **Introductory points.** You will need to be familiar with two types of presentations:

A. Short, 1- to 2-minute, **"bullet" presentations.**

B. More complete, 5- to 6-minute **"formal" presentations.**

The logical flow of the presentation emerges from a good **work-up** and **write-up.** This point emphasizes the importance of using the write-up in preparing for your presentations later in the day or on the next morning. No presentation needs to exceed **6–7 minutes,** even one for a complicated case.

II. **Preparing the data for presentation**

A. **Note card.** A useful adjunct to every write-up, the note card allows the most important parts of the work-up to be summarized, organized, and recorded in a portable, accessible manner. Prepare the note card at the end of the work-up while the case is freshly organized and written. Especially at the beginning of clinical experience, the note card may be used **to present,** unless you are specifically required to present without notes.

B. **Information to note.** At first, it is useful to have a number of facts on the note card. Later, when presenting from memory is less difficult, it is still useful to carry the following information on a note card. (Information that is especially important is marked with an asterisk.)

	Practical points
* **1.** Patient information	Use addressograph plate to stamp top of your card.
* **2.** Introductory sentence	Record necessary information from your write-up.

When providing the information you have obtained to others, provide the data; do not provide conclusions such as "normal." Using conclusions deprives those listening to you of the information they need to draw their own inferences and conclusions.

Donald N. Medearis, Jr., M.D.

* **3.** CC and its duration
  4. HPI
  - **a.** Record salient points, using **single words** that jog your memory and allow you to tell the patient's story as you summarized it.
  - **b.** State pertinent negatives.
  - **c.** State risk factors, positive family history.

  5. PMH — Record only **active problems.**
* **6.** Allergies — Record all and explain type of reaction if drug allergy.
* **7.** Medications — Note **all** (including ethanol and tobacco), with dosages.
  8. ROS — Note **only** significant positives (usually you will have covered these in your HPI).
  9. Physical exam findings
  - **a.** Introductory descriptive sentence.
  - **b.** Vital signs.
  - **c.** Pertinent positive findings only.
* **10.** Laboratory tests — State all **pertinent positive findings.**
* **11.** Problem list — Recorded from the assessment-section plan of the write-up.

The above information should fit onto a 3 × 5-inch index card unless the case is very complicated or you have large writing.

III. Presenting

A. The **bullet presentation** is a *quick,* 1- to 2-minute summary, most often delivered on work rounds in the morning. It is to be considered a **brief, orienting introduction** to those members of the team who do not know the patient at all. Consider the bullet presentation a **summary of the note card** you have prepared: *it is the distillation of your first distillation.*

Outline of the bullet

* **1.** Introductory sentence
* **2.** CC and its duration
  3. HPI

* **4.** Medications
* **5.** Physical exam findings

* **6.** Pertinent positive laboratory tests

  7. Summary

Practical points

Often condensed in a bullet. Include it if your resident wants it; do not drone on. Summarize the HPI in a few sentences.

- **a.** Give the patient's **general condition;** e.g., good, fair, stable, dangerous, comatose.
- **b.** State "**vital signs** stable" or report those that are not.
- **c.** State definitive **positive findings.**

Be brief: if there are laboratory tests your team want to know about, they will ask.

If the case is complicated, give a one- to two-sentence summary.

B. General principles concerning the brief presentation

1. The presentation is a skeleton or framework that allows others to think about the person they are about to meet and the case intelligently.

2. Someone undoubtedly will ask you for anything important that is missing from the bullet. As long as the basic information noted above is given, you have done your job.

3. Speak decisively and distinctly.

4. Mention active and potential problems: this is the time that team members who cover the patients at night hear about them.

Sample bullet

I'll present Mrs. Jones's case formally during attending rounds but to give you all who haven't met her a brief introduction; she's a 55-year-old black seamstress with a history of well-controlled diabetes, hypertension, hyperlipidemia, and rheumatoid arthritis who entered complaining of weakness, cough, and a feverish feeling of 2–3 days' duration. At home, she's been on 80 units of NPH and 15 of CZI insulin per day, takes 50 mg of guanethidine per day, and is on Atromid-S qid.

On physical exam, she's in good condition now with stable vital signs, a temp of 103°F last night, a few rales in her right axilla, but nothing else on her last chest exam. The remainder of her physical exam was unremarkable.

Pertinent labs included a CBC with 12,000 WBCs without a left shift, gram-negative rods on an unspun urine (but no UTI symptoms), and a right lower lobe infiltrate on her chest film. In addition her sputum contained polys and gram-positive diplococci. We think she has pneumoccal pneumonia, and she has begun to defervesce on 500 mg ampicillin IV every 6 hours.

C. The **formal presentation** is essentially a presentation of the note card outlined above (**II.B**).

	Practical points
1. Patient information	If the case is complicated, you may want to interject the phrase "with multiple medical problems."
2. Introductory sentence	
3. CC and its duration	In a presentation, unlike a write-up, **avoid using the patient's words.** Instead, give a description that allows the listeners to focus quickly on the problem at hand.
4. HPI	Present a **succinct** version of the HPI. Give pertinent positive findings from the appropriate ROS section(s). Note pertinent risk factors and family history.
5. PMH	Mention **prior admissions.** Flesh out other active medical problems.
6. Allergies	Note any drug reactions.
7. Medications	State **all present medicines,** with dosages.
8. Positive ROS findings	State only pertinent positives other than those mentioned during the HPI.
9. Physical exam findings	**a. Introductory sentence,** describing appearance and condition.
	b. Vital signs are stated for every patient.
	c. Pertinent positive findings. Some attendings may want you to describe the entire PE system by system, even if normal, but this is unnecessary unless specifically requested.
10. Laboratory tests	**Pertinent positives** from these categories, in this order: CBC, U/A, chemistries, ECG, CXR. ABGs (if done). Pertinent negatives if you believe they are significant.

11. Summary

Give a brief, **two-sentence summary** and then **pause.** The discussion of the case is initiated here so make your summary useful, and make it clear from your voice and expression that you are done. The attending physician will ask you what you and the team did for the patient therapeutically, and will begin discussing specific questions concerning the case (see Part B, I).

B   **Practical Points Concerning Case Presentations**

I. **Areas often discussed during the presentation to the attending.** Rounds with an attending physician ("the visit") are often initiated by the case presentation of the previous night's admission and continue, time permitting, with discussions about the case. The purpose of visit rounds preparation is *not* to be able to anticipate and answer every question you will be asked. Spend the time to reflect about the case, read what you can, and first and foremost understand the pathophysiology. Listed below are some of the frequently discussed areas; although there is rarely time to learn about all of these for each case, choose those subjects you believe are the most pertinent and important to know about for the case in question.

   A. Pathophysiologic mechanisms.

   B. Historical findings and symptoms associated with the disease(s) in question.

   C. Physical findings associated with the disease(s) in question.

   D. Differential diagnosis: other diseases that might present in a similar manner and important differentiating features among these possibilities.

   E. Complications associated with the disease(s) under consideration.

   F. Mechanism of action and side effects of any medications the patient is taking or placed on during this admission.

II. **Caveats of presenting**

   A. Speed of presentation. Do not dawdle, but do not roar through the presentation so quickly that you slur words. A good rule of thumb is to attempt to relax and talk as though explaining a subject to friends.

   B. Tone. Do not read your presentation. This is the most common cause of a monotonic delivery.

   C. Pauses and interruptions. Roll with the punches here; if a discussion ensues while you are presenting, note where you are, listen to and perhaps participate in the digression, and be ready to resume, **repeating** the sentence you last spoke as you begin again. The attending or resident will usually ask you to continue.

   D. Enunciation. Speak precisely. Do not say, for example, "one hundred six" for a temperature of "one-hundred-point-six."

   E. Brevity. The bullet presentation, as noted above, is meant to be brief. However, even the formal presentation should be short enough to maintain the interest of your listeners. Up to 6–7 minutes is a reasonable amount of time to expect people to listen; longer, and you will begin to lose your audience.

   F. Condensation. When it is necessary to detail one or two problems, it becomes necessary as well simply to mention other issues that you may have wished to elaborate on. Condensing the presentation is preferable to making it too long. Describe problems in further detail only in response to your audience's queries.

   G. Omissions. You should describe only positive and negative findings pertinent to the differential diagnoses you are entertaining. In other words, purposefully omit details that are not relevant to the "argument" you are constructing.

   H. Physical exam findings. It is natural at all stages of clinical experience, especially at the beginning, to have equivocal physical findings arise. Point out your

Great science simplifies as it progresses;   rather than add detail.
new concepts ought to give clarity   **Francis D. Moore, M.D.**

findings, and if others have disagreed or differed, simply state, "Another observer thought. . . ."

I. **Concluding.** At the end of the history, physical exam, and laboratory data presentations, summarize the case in one to two sentences for your listeners, focusing on the problem that is most relevant. For example, "In summary, Mrs. Jones is a 55-year-old black woman with a history of diabetes, hypertension, hyperlipidemia, and rheumatoid arthritis who presented last night with a probable pneumococcal pneumonia."

J. **Hospital course.** If the patient has been in the hospital for any length of time, most attending physicians will discuss certain features of the case before they ask about the patient's hospital course. It is reasonable to ask the attending at the end of your presentation whether he or she would like to hear what the patient's hospital course has been. For patients with multiple **active** problems, describe the hospital course in a problem-oriented manner; for example, "First, with respect to the patient's pneumonia. . . . Second, with respect to her elevated blood glucose on admission. . . .," and so on.

K. **Refutations by the bedside.** You will sometimes present by the bedside, and you will almost always see the patient after you present. Patients often refute the stories being told about them, or correct them in major or minor ways. This is not a personal attack; it happens frequently to everyone caring for patients, and it may provide a valuable new clue. Since you are at an advantage, having heard the patient's story previously, try to decipher what the patient has corrected. How was he or she misunderstood originally? Then consider any implications the refutation has for the way in which you have considered the case. Above all, do not panic, and do not argue with the patient.

Selected Summaries of Disease Pathophysiology

Most of us do not know our pathophysiology as well as we should, and often what we do know is not organized in a way that will allow us to apply it easily in patient work-ups. This is primarily because most pathophysiology courses attempt to cover more material than the student is able to assimilate in the time provided. As a result, the student is left without a clear sense of what should be learned first and what can be picked up gradually. The student who masters the basic material presented here early in his or her clinical career will be at an advantage both in ward performance and in the ability to learn further information in a useful way.

Remember the following clinical aphorisms: (1) **common diseases occur commonly,** and (2) **an uncommon presentation of a common disease is more likely than a common manifestation of an uncommon disease.** Both of these concepts are embodied in the familiar clinical saw, "When you hear hoofbeats, think of horses, not zebras."

Part II presents brief summaries of the pathophysiology, clinical manifestations, and differential diagnoses of about 50 of the diseases that you will often encounter on the wards. The information in these entries has been culled principally from three sources: *Harvey's Principles and Practice of Internal Medicine, Cecil and Loeb's Textbook of Medicine,* and *Harrison's Principles of Internal Medicine* (see References).

Our treatment is certainly not a substitute for the comprehensive discussions of the same diseases in these textbooks, but it will provide a general overview and a starting point from which you can move to the major textbooks and the literature.

In order to make this material most useful, we have emphasized those aspects of disease pathophysiology and clinical manifestations that are often discussed in teaching rounds. For those diseases in which comparison to another disease is a central didactic issue, we have presented the clinical manifestations side by side in tables. For those diseases in which pathophysiology is particularly important, we have selected those aspects of the pathophysiology with which the student should be most familiar.

Most serious errors made by physicians are the result of their being unable or unwilling to consider the possibilities that they are misinformed, uninformed, or incorrect. If the patient's history and physical fail to fit neatly into some diagnostic niche, it may be that the history is incomplete, the physical incorrect, or the physician unaware of the correct niche. The patient who refuses to get better despite intensive and expensive therapy may have been treated for the wrong problem and/or, worse yet, may be toxic from the medications. Maimonides was correct: "Teach thy tongue to say I do not know and thou shall progress."

Marshall A. Wolf, M.D.

12

Cardiovascular Diseases

Ischemic Heart Disease: Angina Pectoris and Myocardial Infarction

I. **Definitions**

A. **Angina pectoris.** Clinical syndrome of pain or discomfort in chest and adjacent areas caused by relative myocardial ischemia. By definition, **transient** and **reversible.**

B. **Myocardial infarction. Irreversible** damage to heart muscle that occurs when myocardium is subjected to prolonged ischemia.

II. **Pathophysiology.** Angina pectoris and myocardial infarction are part of a continuum of responses resulting from myocardial oxygen demand exceeding oxygen supply.

Coronary blood flow and the arteriovenous (AV) oxygen difference determine the supply of oxygen to heart muscle. The heart extracts a large percentage of oxygen from coronary arterial blood (large AV oxygen difference); thus, the major determinant of myocardial oxygen supply is **coronary blood flow.** Myocardial oxygen demand is a function of **heart rate, ventricular wall tension,** and the **intrinsic contractile state of the myocardium.** Wall tension is proportional to arterial blood pressure and ventricular volume and inversely proportional to wall thickness. Note that exertion, the major cause of myocardial ischemia, increases each of these determinants of myocardial oxygen demand, and thus myocardial oxygen demand may exceed a limited oxygen supply in patients with coronary artery disease.

One of the more challenging tasks for a physician is to make a *diagnosis of angina pectoris* on the basis of the history. In addition to Levine's sign (in describing the pain the patient clenches his/her fist and places it over the sternum), there are several other less well-known clues:

1. The discomfort of angina pectoris rarely occurs superior to the angle of the jaw or inferior to the umbilicus.
2. If the patient can identify the site of discomfort with his/her index finger it is rarely angina.

Eugene Braunwald, M.D.

Concerning *aortic dissection:* the pain of aortic dissection is characterized most poignantly by its severity and often most aptly by the patient who complains of an internal tearing or ripping. In contradistinction to the pain of myo-cardial ischemia, the patient with aortic dissection often appears restless and agitated in an effort to relieve his or her pain.

Eve E. Slater, M.D.

Edema doesn't always need a diuretic. Right heart failure may require a high filling pressure to maintain output— and edema may reflect a desirable pressure. *Look at the neck veins and decide.*

Cecil H. Coggins, M.D.

III. Clinical manifestations and differential diagnosis

A. Angina. Diagnosis is best made by history.

1. Symptom dimensions

a. Location	Most frequently substernal. May also be in neck, lower jaw, arm or hand areas (especially left arm, ulnar aspect), with or without chest symptoms. Precordial area alone (e.g., left sub-mammary, over heart) **uncommon.**
b. Quality	Often characterized as "discomfort," not "pain." May be described as heavy, tight, squeezing, bandlike, viselike, oppressive, choking, or smothering. Descriptions such as "knifelike," "stabbing," or "cutting" rarely reflect angina.
c. Quantity	Mild to moderate severity; often patients "must" stop whatever they are doing. May seem less bothersome after patients exert themselves for a while ("warm-up" phenomenon). Occurs in crescendo-decrescendo pattern, not of sudden onset or dissipation.
d. Chronology	Patient can usually date month and sometimes even day of onset. Typical attack 1–3 minutes; almost always less than 10 and greater than 1 minute.
e. Setting	Related to exertion or emotion. Cold weather, large meal also may precipitate. Common for angina to occur soon after awakening; shaving or washing may precipitate. Arm exercise may provoke more angina than leg exercise.
f. Aggravating-alleviating factors	Aggravated by emotion, exercise, cold, food; occasionally also by recumbency (angina decubitus). Alleviated by rest, cessation of activity, and often by nitroglycerin. If emotionally precipitated, relieved by relaxation.
g. Associated symptoms	Dyspnea commonly. Nausea, dizziness, diaphoresis sometimes. Palpitation, loss of consciousness **rare** (unless angina is related to arrhythmia).

2. PMH. HTN, tobacco use, DM, lipid disorders, obesity.

3. FHx. H/O ASHD, MI, angina; H/O premature death in male relatives.

4. DDx. The two types of thoracic pain most difficult to differentiate from angina are musculoskeletal and gastrointestinal pain.

a. Musculoskeletal. Usually **persists** for 1 or more hours; often worse at **end of day;** relieved by positional changes, heat; often sharp in quality. Localized (point) tenderness may be present on PE.

b. Gastrointestinal. Not related to exertion, but may be related to anxiety; often related to **meals;** may last up to several hours; relieved by bowel movement, antacid, eructation, position.

Note: GI pain may be relieved by nitroglycerin or calcium channel blockers (e.g., esophageal spasm) and may even be accompanied by ECG changes. Also, GI pain may precipitate anginal pain, or patient may have both GI disease and angina.

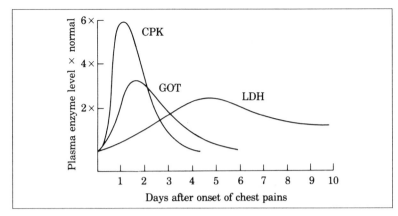

Fig. 12-1. Effect of myocardial infarction on serum enzyme levels.

B. Myocardial infarction. Diagnosis depends on meeting two of three criteria: (1) typical pain, (2) ECG changes, and (3) serum enzyme changes.

   1. Clinical manifestations

   a. Symptoms. Pain most common symptom, often accompanied by nausea, vomiting (classically if MI is **inferior**); diaphoresis, giddiness, anxiety. Preexisting and often worsening angina by history. Approximately 15–20% infarcts painless; painless infarcts more common in diabetics and aged.

   Signs: Associated with pain may be anxiety or, if more extensive myocardial damage, signs of pulmonary edema, shock. Precordium often quiet; S_4, S_3 may be heard, as may soft systolic murmur of MR. Mild fever in first 2–3 days is common.

   b. ECG changes. Appear soon after pain begins.

   Sequence of evolution: (S-T segment elevation, T wave inversion, development of Q waves).

   c. Serum enzyme changes (see Fig. 12-1). Note that the CPK isoenzyme specific to cardiac muscle (**CPK-MB**) is released when damage occurs to the myocardium. This marker is thus a more specific indication of myocardial damage than the unfractionated CK value.

Congestive Heart Failure

I. Definition. Clinical syndrome that results from the inability of the heart to achieve a cardiac output capable of supplying sufficient oxygen to the metabolizing tissues.

II. Etiology. The table below divides the causes of congestive heart failure (CHF) syndrome into six etiologies that tend to lead to CHF by distinct and different pathophysiologic mechanisms. The second column of the table lists the most common event leading to the given etiology of CHF. The last column lists the usual diagnostic route for the disease process in question. *Note that systemic hypertension, valvular heart disease, myocardial disease, and pericardial disease are the subjects of subsequent tables in this chapter.*

	Etiology	Pathophysiology	Most common causes	Usual diagnostic methods
A.	Systemic hypertension (HTN)	↑ Cardiac work load (secondary to ↑ afterload)	Essential HTN	**PE.** ↑ BP and systemic signs of HTN disease (e.g., fundoscopic, renal changes)
B.	Valvular heart disease	↑ Cardiac work load (secondary to ↑ volume or pressure work)	Aortic stenosis; aortic insufficiency; mitral regurgitation; mitral stenosis	Presence of significant murmur(s)
				Specific CV exam findings
				Echocardiography and cardiac catheterization
C.	Myocardial disease	↓ Myocardial contractile function (most cardiomyopathies); or ↓ diastolic filling secondary to ↓ ventricular compliance (e.g., infiltrative processes)	Hypertrophic cardiomyopathy (e.g., HOCM) Primary cardiomyopathy (e.g., viral, alcoholic, postpartum), usually hypodynamic (congestive) type Infiltrative cardiomyopathy (e.g., sarcoid, amyloid), usually restrictive type	**PE.** Congestive (hypodynamic) vs. hypertrophic cardiomyopathies Evidence of systemic disease (e.g., sarcoid, hemochromatosis, connective tissue disease, amyloidosis) **Lab.** Echocardiography; radionuclide ventriculography (RVG); cardiac catheterization; myocardial biopsy
D.	Pericardial disease	↓ Diastolic ventricular filling (causes a fixed restriction in cardiac output)	Viral; traumatic; radiation-induced TB or uremia associated constrictive disease	**PE.** Constrictive pericarditis: signs of RHF (edema, ascites, ↑ venous pressure, hepatomegaly); signs of small quiet heart; CXR may show triangular-shaped heart, calcium in pericardium **Lab.** Echocardiography; cardiac catheterization; characteristic pressure tracings
E.	Pulmonary HTN	↑ Cardiac work load secondary to ↑ pulmonary (right-sided) resistance	Primary pulmonary HTN Pulmonary embolism (acute or chronic) Left heart disease (↑ pulmonary venous pressure) Parenchymal lung disease (e.g., COPD)	**PE.** Signs of RV overload and ↑ pulmonary pressures: parasternal lift; prominent JVP a wave; v wave if tricuspid regurgitation (TR); ↑ intensity P$_2$; murmurs of pulmonic insufficiency (PI) or TR.

Etiology	Pathophysiology	Most common causes	Usual diagnostic methods
			Peripheral signs of RHF: hepatomegaly; edema; pulsatile liver (if TR present)
			Lab. Echocardiography; radionuclide ventriculogram (RVG); right-sided and pulmonary artery catheterization
F. High output states and miscellaneous causes	↑ Workload (secondary to ↑ metabolic demands)	Thyrotoxicosis; anemia **Note:** Underlying disease of heart usually present	**PE.** Search for systemic disease, such as: **Thyrotoxicosis:** hyperactive heart; wide pulse pressure; atrial fibrillation **Anemia:** rapid pulse; hyperactive heart; signs of peripheral vasodilatation **AV fistula:** history of prior surgery; presence of continuous bruit in abnormal location

III. **Exacerbations of CHF.** Often CHF episode is precipitated by some slight change in the baseline compensated state of the patient. This generally occurs secondary to:

Common examples

A. ↓ Myocardial function   ↓ Digoxin (e.g., patient forgets dose), alcohol, new onset arrhythmia, MI

B. ↑ Cardiac work load   ↑ Salt intake ("too much chicken soup"), ↓ Lasix, ↑ activity, infection

Systemic Hypertension

I. **Definitions.** The definition of hypertension is arbitrary, but is at present based on studies defining the relationship between systolic and diastolic pressures and cardiovascular morbidity and mortality rates. Using the blood pressure levels obtained from these studies, hypertensive patients may be diagnosed as:

Women at any age > 160/95
Men above age 45 > 140/95
Men below age 45 > 130/90

It is worth pointing out that a clear impact on cardiovascular mortality by blood pressure control has been demonstrated principally in patients with initial diastolic pressures > 105 mm Hg.

Malignant hypertension is defined as elevated pressures (usually in the > 200/140 range) with evidence of papilledema.

Remember that 97–98% of hypertension is **essential** (idiopathic).

II. **Clinical manifestations.** Findings associated with hypertension vary; the degree of symptomatology and physical exam evidence of hypertension is roughly correlated with the degree of blood pressure elevation.

A. Symptoms may include headache, nosebleed, palpitations, vertigo, tinnitus, or even nervousness.

1. With **increasing pressures,** cardiovascular dysfunction may become apparent as orthopnea, dyspnea, anginal symptoms, and even frank pulmonary edema. Ocular fatigue, decreased visual activity, visual blurring, and occipital headaches may all be present.

2. With **high pressures,** severe headaches may develop, with associated visual impairment, drowsiness, and even encephalopathic changes. Transient paresthesias, CVAs may also appear with higher pressures.

B. Signs are classically described in the cardiovascular, visual (retinal), and nervous systems.

1. **Cardiac** findings due to hypertension may arise from hypertrophic myocardial changes in response to increased afterload. Possible findings include an LV heave, laterally displaced and sustained apex beat, and fourth heart sound.

   With progressive cardiac disease due to HTN, cardiomegaly may develop, with associated murmurs of AI and/or MR as well as with signs of LV failure (e.g., third heart sound, pulsus alternans).

2. **Retinal** changes follow a progression based on the severity and duration of the elevation in blood pressure. Ophthalmologists order these changes in a specific, numerical system for grading retinal changes.

   a. **Earlier retinal changes** include arterial narrowing and variations in caliber of the arterioles. Hard exudates may appear, as may flame-shaped hemorrhages.

   b. With **higher blood pressures,** an increase in the number of hemorrhages may occur, and soft exudates appear.

   c. **Papilledema,** the most severe retinal change, defines malignant hypertension.

3. **CNS** changes include transient weakness or numbness, paresthesias, and an increasing incidence of cerebral thrombotic or hemorrhagic events.

   Hypertensive encephalopathy occurs with very high blood pressures and is characterized by transient, focal CNS deficits, severe headache, visual disturbances, and even convulsions, stupor, and coma.

C. Laboratory abnormalities

1. **Urinalysis** may reveal proteinuria; hematuria can occur, usually with higher pressures.

2. **Chemistries** may show evidence of renal disease, with increased BUN and creatinine values.

3. **ECG** may show increased voltage consistent with LVH, as well as "strain" patterns of T wave flattening or inversion, especially in lateral leads.

4. **CXR** may show cardiomegaly, with LV prominence. Dilatation or tortuosity of the ascending aorta may be a prominent feature as well.

Myocardial Disease

I. **Definition.** Disease in which the clinical presentation is due to dysfunction of the myocardium as a result of a process that primarily affects the myocardial tissue. Classically, myocardial changes due to systemic or pulmonary hypertension, ischemic heart disease, and valvular disease are **excluded** from this group of myocardial disorders.

II. **Congestive and hypertrophic cardiomyopathy.** The table below compares the two most common of the three types of cardiomyopathy. The third type, **restrictive** cardiomyopathy, is not discussed.

	Congestive (hypodynamic) cardiomyopathy	Hypertrophic obstructive cardiomyopathy (HOCM)
A. Common etiologies	Infective (viral, bacterial)	Familial (autosomal dominant trait)
	Metabolic (puerperal, thyroid disease, hemochromatosis)	
	Alcoholic	
	Systemic disease (SLE)	
B. Clinical manifestations	Viral illness, recent pregnancy, alcoholism, etc.	FHx heart disease; often asymptomatic
	CHF (e.g., dyspnea, orthopnea); may be severe	Angina, dyspnea, syncope
C. PE	Sinus tachycardia	LV lift
	Pulsus alternans	Bisferiens carotid pulse ("spike and dome" morphology)
	Diffuse PMI	
	S_3, MR murmur	Bifid-trifid apical impulse
	Prominent v wave with JVP	SEM, which *increases* with Valsalva or upon standing.
		S_4 and, if MR present, S_3
D. ECG	Atrial arrhythmias	LVH with strain
	Q waves and abnormal QRS complexes	LAD
	Conduction defects	"Bizarre" Q waves
	Ventricular arrhythmias	WPW syndrome
		Conduction defects
E. CXR	Cardiomegaly, may be massive	Signs of LVH
	Pulmonary congestion	
F. ECHO	Large, poorly contracting heart	Asymmetric ventricular hypertrophy (e.g., septal hypertrophy)

Pericardial Disease

I. **Definition.** Cardiovascular dysfunction due to acute or chronic changes involving the pericardium, either from a primary disease process or as a manifestation of systemic illness.

II. **Acute and chronic pericarditis.** Pericarditis is classically divided into acute and chronic forms because, as the table shows, acute and chronic pericarditis have very different clinical presentations and courses.

	Acute pericarditis	Chronic (constrictive) pericarditis
A. Common etiologies	Idiopathic	Often idiopathic
	Viral (Coxsackie B)	Occasionally H/O acute pericarditis

	Acute pericarditis	**Chronic (constrictive) pericarditis**
	Bacterial	
	TB	
	Uremia	
	Post-MI	
B. Clinical manifestations	Antecedent URI	Dyspnea
	Sharp, substernal chest pain, often with left supraclavicular radiation	Edema
		Ascites
	↑ Pain with supine position	Signs of CHF
	↓ Pain with sitting, leaning forward	
	Malaise, constitutional symptoms	
	Fever	Pulsus paradoxus
	Myalgias	Venous distension
	Pericardial friction rub	Prominent JVP *a* wave and rapid y wave descent
	± Pericardial effusion	Pericardial knock in early diastole
		Kussmaul's sign
		Hepatomegaly
		Ascites
		Edema
C. Lab	Mild to moderate leukocytosis	↓ Serum albumin
	↑ ESR	Lymphopenia
D. ECG	S-T segment elevation without QRS changes	Low voltage
		Irregular P wave
	Supraventricular arrhythmias (e.g., APBs, PAT, atrial fibrillation or flutter)	Atrial fibrillation
		Nonspecific S-T and T wave changes
E. CXR	± Enlarged cardiac silhouette	Small heart
		± Calcium in pericardium
		Irregular or triangularly shaped heart
		Dilated SVC
F. ECHO	Effusion ± pericardial thickening	Pericardial thickening
		Small ventricular chamber size
		Enlarged atrial chamber size

Peripheral Vascular Disease

I. **Definition.** Acute or chronic changes in the arterial or venous vasculature that lead to alterations in the normal physiologic functions of blood supply.

II. **Arterial disease.** The common clinical presentations of acute and chronic arterial vascular disease are compared in the table below.

	Acute arterial disease	**Chronic arterial disease**
A. Etiology	Inadequate distal oxygenation secondary to occlusion by embolus (90% originate from heart)	Inadequate distal oxygenation secondary to arterial lumen compromise by atherosclerotic plaque/stenosis
B. Symptoms	Pain, paresthesias, numbness	Intermittent claudication (muscle ischemia)
		Chronic rest pain (later stages) ± paresthesias
C. Signs	Sudden onset: pale extremity; loss of pulse; ↓ temperature distal to occlusion	↓ Or absent peripheral pulse(s)
		↓ Temperature distal to occlusion
		Bruit(s) over involved area
		Feet: pallor on elevation; delayed capillary blush on lowering to dependent position; rubor on dependency
		Trophic skin changes: ↓ hair and/or nail growth; less reliable signs
		Ulcers: inferior to malleoli; toes most common site
D. Risk factors	Mural thrombi: atrial fibrillation-arrhythmias S/P recent MI; chronic CHF, cardiomyopathy; H/O endocarditis	Diabetes mellitus
		Cigarette smoking
		Hypertension
		Obesity
		Hyperlipidemia
E. Common site(s)	Narrowed areas and bifurcations: femoral artery–profunda femoris junction; aortoiliac junction	Superficial femoral involved in vast majority of patients
		Aortoiliac, popliteal areas also common

III. **Venous disease.** The common clinical presentations of acute and chronic venous disease are compared in the table below.

	Acute venous disease	**Chronic venous disease**
A. Etiology	Impaired venous return (VR) secondary to **thrombophlebitis** (also external venous compression, trauma)	Impaired VR secondary to thrombotic disruption of venous vessels and valves
B. Symptoms	Thrombophlebitis may be asymptomatic	Aching pain after standing or sitting
	Pain, aching, tenderness over muscles	

	Acute venous disease	Chronic venous disease
C. Signs	Superficial venous distension	Thickened, discolored (brown) overlying skin
	Swelling, edema	Secondary varicosities
	Cyanosis	Pruritis
	Measurable difference in calf circumference	**Ulcers:** anterior and superior to lateral malleoli
D. Risk factors	Conditions leading to venous stasis (S/P MI, post-op, hemiplegia, etc.)	Pregnancy
		Ascites
	Hypercoaguable states (e.g., polycythemia vera)	Abdominal tumor
E. Common site(s)	Deep and superficial veins of lower extremities	Excessive weight or height
		Deep and superficial veins of lower extremities

IV. Definitions of related syndromes

A. Raynaud's disease. Symptom complex of pain and pallor in fingers and/or toes following exposure to cold or emotional upset.

B. Raynaud's phenomenon. Symptom complex of Raynaud's disease found in association with systemic disease (e.g., collagen vascular diseases).

C. Leriche's syndrome. Impotence and bilateral buttock and thigh pain due to aortoiliac atherosclerotic disease.

D. Thromboangiitis obliterans (*Buerger's* disease). Vascular disease characterized by occlusion of small-medium arteries below the elbow and knee, which may lead to necrosis of the digits of hands and feet. Most commonly seen in young Jewish males who are heavy smokers. Thrombophlebitis often coexists.

Mitral Valve Disease

I. **Definition.** Alterations in the integrity or normal functioning of the mitral valve or its associated structures that lead to alterations in normal cardiovascular physiology.

II. **Mitral stenosis and mitral regurgitation.** The table below compares some common features of mitral stenosis and mitral regurgitation. Unless otherwise stated, mitral regurgitation refers to the **chronic** lesion.

	Mitral stenosis	Mitral regurgitation
A. Pathophysiology	Rheumatic heart disease (RHD): 50%, will give history of rheumatic fever	RHD; congenital; mitral prolapse; (ruptured chordae or papillary muscle dysfunction causes acute MR)
B. Clinical manifestations	DOE; pulmonary edema; hemoptysis; fatigue; reactive pulmonary hypertension; right heart failure	In **chronic** MR fatigue, DOE **gradually** appear; if **acute,** sudden onset of CHF symptoms
C. Heart sounds	Loud S_1; opening snap	Diminished S_1; S_3 due to volume overload
D. Murmur	Localized near apex; onset at opening snap (middiastolic) of a low-pitched rumbling. Presystolic accentuation of murmur if	Loudest over PMI; pansystolic; blowing; midpitched; radiating to axilla

	Mitral stenosis	Mitral regurgitation
	normal sinus rhythm is present. Graham-Steell murmur of pulmonary insufficiency may be present	
E. X-ray	Straight left heart border, large LA, RV; mitral valve calcification; Kerley B-lines; prominence of upper lung field vasculature	LV and LA enlargement; minimal pulmonary congestion if chronic.
F. ECG	Broad, notched P waves; axis normal or right axis deviation (RAD); atrial fibrillation common	LAD; tall P waves, sometimes notched; atrial fibrillation common

Aortic Valve Disease

I. **Definition.** Alterations in the integrity or normal functioning of the aortic valve and/or the aortic infravalvular or supravalvular structures that lead to alterations in the normal physiology of the cardiovascular system.

II. **Aortic stenosis and aortic insufficiency.** The table below compares some common features of aortic stenosis and aortic insufficiency.

	Aortic stenosis	Aortic insufficiency
A. Pathophysiology	Congenital lesion, (e.g., bicuspid valve); rheumatic heart disease; calcific aortic stenosis	RHD; endocarditis; congenital; dissecting aneurysm; syphilis; inflammatory diseases; subvalvular structural disease
B. Clinical manifestations	CHF, angina, and syncope, are three main symptoms; presence of **any one** indicates need for surgical therapy	CHF or angina late in course; may be asymptomatic or have subtle decreases in exercise tolerance for long period of time
C. Heart sounds	A_2 normal or decreased in calcific AS (may be *increased* in congenital AS); S_4 gallop	A_2 normal or decreased; S_3 gallop
D. Murmur	Right second ICS parasternally or at apex; midsystolic; harsh, rough; transmitted to neck. **Key** to diagnosis of significant AS is a carotid pulse with decreased upstroke and volume (*pulsus tardus et parvus*)	Left sternal border in third to fourth ICS; begins after A_2 and ends before S_1; blowing, faint ("wind whistling in the trees")
E. X-ray	± LV enlargement; prominent ascending aorta; calcified valve in calcific form	Large (perhaps very large) LV
F. ECG	LV hypertrophy	LV hypertrophy; LAD

Peptic Ulcer Disease

I. **Definition.** An ulcer found in the esophagus, stomach, or duodenum caused directly or indirectly by gastric secretions.

II. **Pathophysiology**

A. Pathogenesis unclear; leading theories involve both **gastric hypersecretion** and **mucosal breakdown**. Duodenal ulcer disease may be quite different from gastric ulcer disease.

B. Duodenal ulcer patients as a group secrete twice the acid of normals, but there is a large overlap between the two groups.

C. Mucosal junctions (esophagus-stomach; pylorum-duodenum; fundus-antrum) are most commonly affected sites.

D. Pain may be result of nerve irritation by acid, or increased tone in duodenum and antrum.

E. **Zollinger-Ellison syndrome.** Gastric hypersecretion associated with gastrin-secreting islet tumors of the pancreas.

III. **Clinical manifestations**

A. **Symptoms and signs.** Gnawing, burning pain in midepigastrium and esopha-

---

The patient with right-upper quadrant pain, hematuria, fever, and diarrhea may also have Crohn's disease (the gallstone-kidney stone-Crohn's complex).

Multiple organ involvement often suggests systemic disease.
Z. Myron Falchuk, M.D.

The terms "acute abdomen" and "surgical abdomen" are unfortunate, misleading, and should be abandoned. Not only are these labels misconstrued by many to be tantamount to the need for urgent surgical intervention, but they also convey the erroneous suggestion that the goal to be sought in a patient with the recent onset of abdominal pain is solely that of identification of the condition as acute and surgical, or nonsurgical. Since the most catastrophic of abdominal conditions, such as strangulating intestinal obstruction or impending rupture of an aortic aneurysm, often have surprisingly mild symptoms for 24 or even 48 hours with the subtlest of findings on examination, the diagnosis will be missed if the physician is antici-

pating a patient with boardlike rigidity who is writhing in pain. Conversely, conditions in which operation may be interdicted, such as acute pancreatitis or pulmonary infarction, may cause impressive abdominal pain, rigidity, and absent peristaltic sounds (although the presence or absence of peristaltic sounds and the character of the sounds are of little value and are often misleading). A careful and time-consuming history and physical examination directed at reaching a specific diagnosis will be far more rewarding than attempts to categorize the condition as surgical or nonsurgical, and cannot be replaced by currently available laboratory tests.
William Silen, M.D.

gus, nausea, vomiting.

B. Lab findings. ± GI bleeding, ± gastric hypersecretion. UGI series may show ulcer craters or gastritis with ↑ folds, esophagitis.

C. Complications. Hemorrhage, perforation, penetration into adjacent organs, pyloric obstruction, gastric malignancy, chronic pain.

IV. Differential diagnosis

A. Peptic ulcer disease (PUD) must be distinguished from gastritis, pancreatitis, diverticulitis, appendicitis, inflammatory bowel disease, and gastric carcinoma. Dx is made on basis of Hx, endoscopy, x-rays, secretory study, biopsy, cytology.

B. Gastric vs. duodenal ulcers

Feature	Gastric ulcer	Duodenal ulcer
Usual site	Lesser curvature	Duodenal bulb
Sex predilection	1 : 1 male-female	4 : 1 male-female
Pain	After meals	Relieved by meals
Pathology	May be malignant	Rarely malignant
Gastric acid	Low or normal	Hypersecretion
Vomiting	Common	Uncommon

Cholecystitis

I. Definition. Inflammation of the gallbladder usually secondary to obstruction of cystic duct by a calculus.

II. Pathophysiology

A. Gallstones present in 15% of Americans age 55–65. Predominance in American Indians, patients with regional enteritis and DM. Male-female ratio 1 : 2.

B. Cholesterol stones composed of cholesterol, phospholipids, conjugated bile salts. Bile salts in water form micelles, which solubilize cholesterol and phospholipids, so stone formation depends on relative proportion of all three constituents. Cholesterol stones (>75% cholesterol by weight) account for 75% of stones in U.S.; **pigment stones** (<10% cholesterol) account for 20% and contain mostly calcium bilirubinate and unconjugated bilirubin.

C. Stages of cholesterol gallstone formation

1. Chemical stage. Secretion of bile supersaturated with cholesterol occurs during fasting.

2. Crystallization stage. Precipitation and crystallization in gallbladder.

3. Growth stage. Coalescence of microscopic stones into macroscopic stones.

III. Clinical manifestations. Onset of classic attack often follows meal of fried or fatty foods. Steady, sometimes severe pain in epigastrium may be accompanied by nausea, vomiting, jaundice, fever. Pain may radiate to infrascapular area and subside spontaneously after 12–18 hours. Lab shows ↑ WBC, ↑ serum bilirubin (1–4 mg/dl). X-ray studies (including IV cholangiography, oral cholecystography) often useful, although most stones are not radioopaque.

Choledocholithiasis develops in over 15% of cholelithiasis patients. *Charcot's triad* (pain, fever, jaundice) is characteristic of an acutely obstructed duct.

IV. Differential diagnosis. Pancreatitis, perforated peptic ulcer, appendicitis, carcinoma, hepatitis must be ruled out. Dx on basis of Hx, x-ray and ultrasound studies.

Gastrointestinal Bleed

I. **Definition.** Acute or chronic blood loss from any point in the GI tract, resulting in hematemesis or hematochezia.

II. **Pathophysiology**

A. Common causes of **upper GI bleeds**

1. Erosive gastritis or duodenitis

2. Duodenal or gastric ulcers

3. Esophageal varices

B. Common causes of **lower GI bleeds**

1. Hemorrhoids

2. Ulcerative colitis or Crohn's disease

3. Colorectal carcinoma

4. Benign rectal polyps

5. Bleeding diverticuli

6. Angiodysplasia

III. **Clinical manifestations and differential diagnosis.** Key is to determine *site* of bleeding: Hx important (alcohol? drug? PUD?); endoscopy and x-ray studies very valuable. Angiography may be required.

IV. **Signs and symptoms**

Signs and symptoms	Clinical correlation
A. Red blood per rectum	Either lower GI lesion or massive upper GI lesion with fast transit time
B. Hematemesis; blood in gastric aspirate	Bleeding proximal to ligament of Treitz; "coffee grounds" in aspirate suggest bleeding has stopped
C. Low hematocrit	Suggests that bleeding began at least 12 hours ago; hemodilution may take 24 hours or more
D. Sx of shock (tachycardia, hypotension, clammy skin)	Loss of 20–30% of total blood volume if Sx present when patient upright; 50% loss if present while patient recumbent
E. Guaiac-positive stools	Loss of > 10 ml blood per day; continuous occult bleeding suggests malignancy; intermittent bleeding suggests benign lesions (polyps, hemorrhoids)
F. ↑ BUN with normal creatinine	Result of recent GI bleed and digestion of intraintestinal blood.

Acute Viral Hepatitis

I. **Definition**

A. **Hepatitis A.** *Infectious* hepatitis associated with fecal-oral transmission, fecal shedding of 27 nmol particle (?RNA virus), and incubation period of 15–40 days.

B. **Hepatitis B.** *Serum* hepatitis associated with transmission by way of parenteral inoculation (often infected blood products), shedding of 42 nmol Dane particle (DNA virus) with Hb_sAg surface antigen (detectable in > 80% of patients with acute infection), and incubation period of 50–160 days. Some cases progress to chronic hepatitis. Commonly presents in IV drug abusers and homosexual men.

C. **Non-A, non-B hepatitis.** Posttransfusion hepatitis with incubation period of 15–180 days causing clinical picture similar to that of hepatitis B but not associated with A or B viral type.

II. **Clinical manifestations.** The presentation of acute viral hepatitis is similar for all three types.

A. **Prodrome.** Lasts 2–14 days. Common findings are anorexia, nausea, vomiting, malaise, "flu" Sx, fever, enlarged and tender liver, abnormal SGOT, SGPT, LDH.

B. **Icteric phase.** Jaundice, ↑ lymphocytes (some abnormal), intensification of Sx, dark urine are found. Increased PT may signal hepatocellular necrosis. Circulating Hb_sAg is present in hepatitis B.

C. **Convalescent phase-complication.** Gradual resolution. Dangerous complications include fulminant hepatitis (hepatic failure and encephalopathy usually with hepatitis B) and chronic active hepatitis (5–10% of hepatitis B) where biopsy shows "piecemeal necrosis" and Hb_sAg persists.

III. **Differential diagnosis.** Acute viral hepatitis must be distinguished from other viral infections (cytomegalovirus [CMV], herpes simplex virus, Coxsackie virus), cholecystitis, drug reactions. Dx is often made on the basis of serologic detection of specific antigens and antibodies.

Acute Appendicitis

I. **Definition.** Inflammation of the appendix, often secondary to mucosal ulcerations or lumenal obstruction.

II. **Pathophysiology**

A. Most common in patients ages 10–30.

B. Incidence much lower in undeveloped countries (dietary factors?).

C. Appendiceal obstruction often due to fecolith, but also may be caused by kinking, lymphoid swelling, foreign body, or neoplasm. Bacterial infection and lumenal necrosis often follow obstruction.

III. **Clinical manifestations**

A. **Presentation.** Classic picture begins with periumbilical epigastric discomfort first, then anorexia, vomiting, nausea. Within several hours, pain shifts to RLQ, sometimes localized at McBurney's point. Associated findings include fever, left-shifted PMN, constipation, psoas and obturator signs.

B. **Complications.** Perforation (followed by peritonitis) and/or appendiceal abscess formation may occur.

IV. **Differential diagnosis.** Major DDx is appendicitis vs. gastroenteritis vs. mesenteric adenitis. Other possible diagnoses are pelvic inflammatory disease, diverticulitis, Crohn's disease, rupture of ovarian follicle (Mittleschmerz). Diagnosis is made on basis of Hx and PE.

Chronic Inflammatory Bowel Disease (Crohn's Disease and Ulcerative Colitis)

I. **Definition.** Crohn's disease (regional enteritis) is a chronic inflammatory disease of the GI tract (most often terminal ileum and right colon) distinguished by transmural intestinal involvement with skipped areas. Ulcerative colitis is a chronic inflammatory disease (usually involving left more often than right colon) distinguished by destruction of intestinal crypts, continuous involvement, pseudopolyposis, rectal bleeding, and occasional progression to malignancy.

II. **Pathophysiology.** The pathophysiology is unknown: Perhaps multiple etiologies? Same disease? Familial incidences are high.

III. Clinical manifestations and differential diagnosis of Crohn's disease vs. ulcerative colitis

Feature	Crohn's disease	Ulcerative colitis
A. Onset	Gradual	Gradual or abrupt
B. Signs and symptoms	Intermittent crampy abdominal pain, low-grade fever, diarrhea, very little bleeding	Bloody diarrhea, anorexia, urgency, fever, anemia
C. Pathology	Thickened intestine, ulcerated "cobblestone" mucosa, transmural lymphoid hyperplasia, fistulas, noncaseating granulomas	"Crypt abscess" formation, infiltration of lamina propria by inflammatory cells, pseudopolyps
D. Radiologic findings	Ileal narrowing, fuzzy mucosal pattern on barium enema	Straight and narrow colon, loss of haustra, ulcer craters, small polypoid-filling defects
E. Complications	Stricture obstructions, abscess formation, perforation, perirectal fistulas, gallstones, kidney stones	Colonic perforation, toxic megacolon, colonic carcinoma late in course.

Pancreatitis

I. **Definition.** Acute or chronic inflammation of the pancreas.

II. **Pathophysiology**

  A. Acute pancreatitis often secondary to biliary tract disease, alcoholism, or abdominal surgery.

  B. Some attacks may be precipitated by impaction of gallstones in ampulla of Vater, causing release of pancreatic enzymes and tissue necrosis. Edema, hemorrhage, and necrosis are mediated partially by release of trypsin, elastase, phospholipase A, and plasma kinins (↑ vascular permeability) leading to compressive ischemia. Pathologic changes include fat necrosis and formation of pseudocysts and abscesses.

  C. Chronic pancreatitis often secondary to alcoholism. Tissue damage may be due to a variety of factors: protein malnutrition, abnormal bile formation (↑ free bile acids), direct EtOH toxicity, ↑ pancreatic secretion leading to duct obstruction.

III. **Clinical manifestations**

  A. **Acute pancreatitis.** Severe abdominal pain continuing for hours or days; nausea, vomiting, fever, ↓ BP. Abdominal rigidity and rebound tenderness may be present. Ecchymoses on flanks (Grey Turner's sign) or around umbilicus (Cullen's sign) suggest hemorrhage or extensive inflammation. Lab tests show ↑ WBC and elevated serum amylase (sometimes marked).

  B. **Chronic pancreatitis.** Presentation may involve weight loss, glucose intolerance, or recurrent abdominal pain. Symptoms generally similar to those of acute pancreatitis. Serum amylase levels may not be elevated if disease is advanced. X-ray may show pancreatic calcification. Before nitrogen wasting or steatorrhea become obvious, 90% of pancreatic tissue must be destroyed.

IV. **Differential diagnosis**

  A. **Acute pancreatitis** must be distinguished from other causes of abdominal inflammation: cholelithiasis, common duct stones, intestinal obstruction or perforation, ectopic pregnancy, PID, PUD.

  B. **Chronic pancreatitis,** which may be relatively painless, must be distinguished from malabsorption syndromes, diverticuli, pancreatic carcinoma.

  C. **Serum amylase level** is the single most valuable laboratory test in DDx.

II. Clinical manifestations and differential diagnosis of Crohn's disease vs. ulcerative colitis

Feature	Crohn's disease	Ulcerative colitis

14   Genitourinary Diseases

Acute Renal Failure

I. **Definition.** Acute suppression of kidney filtration by function, usually accompanied by oliguria.

II. **Pathophysiology**

   A. **Etiologies**

      1. **Prerenal.** Hemorrhage, septicemia, fluid-electrolyte depletion (leading to ↓ perfusion).

      2. **Postrenal.** Prostatism, tumor obstruction, calculi, congenital anomalies.

      3. **Renal.** Ischemia, toxins, burns, drug reaction, vascular obstruction, glomerulonephritis, intrarenal precipitates.

   B. Damage occurs through direct **nephrotoxicity** (usually involving necrosis of tubular epithelium) and **ischemia** (often secondary to vasomotor nephropathy, the constriction of afferent arterioles).

   C. Although oliguria is common, the volume of urine bears no relation to the degree of functional impairment.

III. **Clinical manifestations.** The presentation of ARF can be divided into two phases.

   A. **Oliguric phase.** Associated findings are ↓ ↓ urine formation (< 20 ml/hr) with rising blood urea and/or serum creatinine levels; anorexia, nausea, vomiting; urine sediment consisting of protein, red cells, epithelial cells, brown granular casts; specific gravity 1.010–1.016; ↓ serum Na^+ (120–130 mEq/L); hyperkalemia; Hct 25–30%; ↑ BUN and creatinine.

   B. **Diuretic phase.** Begins approximately 2 weeks postonset. Gradual ↑ in urine formation to 6–8 L/day, indicating nephron recovery. Continuous for 7–10 days.

IV. **Differential diagnosis of prerenal azotemia vs. intrinsic renal azotemia**

Determination	Prerenal	Renal
Urine osmolality	> 500 mOsm/L	< 350 mOsm/L
Urine: plasma creatinine	> 20	< 10
Urine: plasma urea	> 40	< 20
Urine Na^+	< 20 mEq/L	> 40 mEq/L

Glomerulonephropathies

I. **Definition.** A group of diseases characterized by damage to the renal glomerulus

---

Dehydration in an attempt to reduce pulmonary edema of adult respiratory distress syndrome (ARDS) is a worthy goal, but keep in mind that *the kidney has a right to life too, and its blood flow must be maintained at all costs.* Renal failure doubles the mortality of ARDS. In addition, there is no evidence that maintenance of normal plasma oncotic pressure prevents or treats pulmonary edema caused by abnormal pulmonary vascular wall permeability.

                    Henning Pontoppidan, M.D.

often resulting in abrupt hematuria, proteinuria, and red cell casts in the urine.

II. Pathophysiology

A. Etiologic mechanisms

1. **Immunologic mechanisms**

   a. **Immune complex diseases** are secondary to poststreptococcal and other infectious agents (staphylococcus, pneumococcus, hepatic viruses). SLE and other autoimmune diseases, membranous and membranoproliferative syndromes (cause?), focal glomerulonephritis.

   b. **Antiglomerular basement membrane** diseases, e.g., Goodpasture's syndrome.

2. **Unclear mechanisms** (possibly immunologic). Lipoid nephrosis, amyloidosis, hemolytic uremic syndrome, chronic sclerosing glomerulonephritis, sickle cell disease, lymphomas.

B. Pathophysiologic sequence of poststreptococcal glomerulonephritis

1. Beta-hemolytic streptococci injure mesangial cells in glomerulus.

2. Ag-Ab complexes further injure mesangial and epithelial cells, which proliferate.

3. IgG and C3 deposited in granular pattern on epithelial side of basement membrane.

4. Endocapillary cell proliferation occludes glomerular capillaries and causes kidney to enlarge.

III. Clinical manifestations of poststreptococcal glomerulonephritis. Usually sequence begins with sore throat and fever; in 2–3 weeks, urine becomes smoky, with ↓ volume. Edema of face and ankles. Some weakness, anorexia, H/A, SOB, and azotemia develop. Hypertension (115–120 mm Hg diastolic) is common.

U/A reveals hematuria, proteinuria, and hyaline, granular, and RBC casts. Complications include CHF, severe hypertension, infection. Nephrotic "crisis" occurs, characterized by prostration, abdominal pain, behavioral changes, vomiting, fever. (These Sx may be caused by localized edema of ligament of Treitz.)

IV. Differential diagnosis. The crucial question in DDx is **etiology** of nephrotic syndrome; percutaneous biopsy is often helpful (see Table 14-1).

Chronic Renal Failure

I. Definition. Chronic insufficiency of the renal excretory and regulatory functions leading to uremia.

II. Pathophysiology

A. Etiologies. Primary glomerular disease, hypertension, nephrotoxins, renal vascular disease, pyelonephritis, infectious metabolic diseases (especially DM and gout), obstructive uropathy, congenital diseases (polycystic kidney, tubular acidosis). All result in parenchymal scarring and glomerular hyalinization.

B. Uremia results from nephron loss and decreased GFR (up to 70% of renal tissue may be lost before any change in GFR occurs). Osmotic diuresis leads to dehydration. Inadequate regulation of electrolyte excretion leads to anion-pH abnormalities. Na^+ loss lead to ↓ ECF, causing ↓↓ renal perfusion. Abnormal vitamin D and PTH causes secondary hyperparathyroidism. Decreased nitrogen clearance leads to ↑ serum urea, creatinine, urate. Hypertension and anemia (↓ renal erythropoietin synthesis) gradually develop.

III. Clinical manifestations. Early manifestations include weakness, fatigue, anorexia, nausea. PE may reveal neuropathy. Asymptomatic pericarditis is common. Toxic

psychosis may cause behavior disturbances and coma. Lab findings include azotemia, acidosis (CO_2 15–20 mEq/L) hyperphosphatemia, hyperkalemia, and normochromic normocytic anemia. Urine osmolarity ~ 300–320 mOsm/liter. Gradually, the complications discussed in **II** may develop. In advanced renal disease, there are signs of malnutrition, GI bleeding, yellow-brown skin discoloration, pruritis, and CHF.

IV. Differential diagnosis. The major diagnostic question involves the **etiology** of the renal insufficiency. Some etiologies are reversible (infection, obstruction, drug toxicity, gout), so the clinical picture must be evaluated carefully. A more definitive Dx may be made on the basis of renal biopsy.

Nephrotic Syndrome

I. Definition. Nephrotic syndrome is characterized by:

A. Proteinuria ($\geq$ 3.5 gm/day).

B. Hypoalbuminemia ($\leq$ 300 mg/100 ml).

C. Lipiduria. In addition, hypercholesterolemia ($\geq$ 300 mg/100 ml) and edema are usually present.

II. Pathophysiology

A. Common etiologies

1. **Primary renal diseases.** Lipoid nephrosis; membranous, membranoproliferative, and focal sclerosing glomerulonephritis; renal vein thrombosis; Goodpasture's syndrome.

2. **Nephrotoxins.** Mercury, gold, bismuth.

3. **Systemic illnesses.** SLE, DM, amyloidosis, e.g.

B. Pathophysiologic sequence

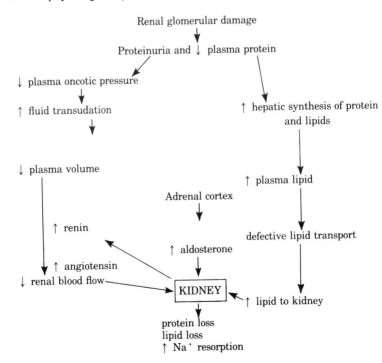

Table 14-1. Features of glomerulonephropathies

Glomerulonephropathy	Light microscopy	Electron microscopy	Immunofluorescence				
			IgG	IgA	IgM	C3	FRA
Primary glomerulonephritis							
Diffuse proliferative, including poststreptococcal	Proliferation of mesangial cells, endothelial cells, and/or epithelial cells	Subepithelial GBM deposits; increased mesangial cells and matrix	Variable and irregular granular deposits along capillary walls and in mesangium	++	v	v	+	v
Focal proliferative	Focal proliferative changes plus increased mesangial cellularity	Mesangial deposits	Segmental granular GBM and mesangial deposits	++	+	+	++	v
Proliferative with crescent formation	Crescent formation from proliferation of epithelial cells filling Bowman's space	Subendothelial deposits along GBM with increased mesangial matrix; proliferating epithelial cells	Diffuse granular or linear deposits involving peripheral capillary loops	++	+	+	+	+
Mesangiocapillary (membranoproliferative)	Proliferation of mesangial cells; increased mesangial matrix; thickening of capillary walls	I. Deposits in mesangium; endothelial cells separated from endothelial cells by mesangial matrix II. Confluent intra-GBM deposits	I. Granular deposit along GBM; C3 alone in mesangium II. Intramembranous deposit in GBM and TBM	++	v	++	+++	v
Membranous	Thickening of capillary wall; subepithelial spikes (silver stain)	Dense subepithelial deposits	Coarse granular deposits along capillary wall	++	v	v	++	v
Chronic, end-stage	Hyalinization of glomeruli	Fibrosis, hyaline deposits	Granular deposits in mesangium	±	±	±	+	±

Systemic disease							
Systemic lupus erythematosus	Variable patterns of minimal changes, mesangial proliferation, focal proliferation, membranous lesions; hematoxylin bodies in capillary loops	Characteristic massive subendothelial, intramembranous, and subepithelial deposits; wire-loop lesions; microtubules in endothelial cells and leukocytes	Variable; granular deposits corresponding to type and location of altered glomeruli	++	+	++	++	+
Diseases of uncertain immunologic cause							
Lipoid nephrosis	No alteration, or minimal lesion of proliferative type	Abnormalities of epithelial cells with smudging of foot processes and obliteration of slit-bore membrane	Minimal irregular clumps in mesangial areas	±	−	±	±	−
Berger's IgA nephropathy	Segmental to diffuse mesangial proliferation and increase in mesangial matrix	Deposits in mesangium	Granular deposits in mesangium	+	++	++	++	+

FRA = fibrin-fibrinogen–related antigen; v = variable; GBM = glomerular basement membrane; TBM = tubular basement membrane.
Source: From M. Krupp and M. Chatton, *Current Medical Diagnosis and Treatment 1981.* Los Altos, Calif.: Lange, 1981. P. 532.

III. **Clinical manifestations.** Besides the classic Sx of edema, abdominal protuberance, anorexia, and pallor, common manifestations include retinal sheens, hypertension, and growth retardation.

IV. **Differential diagnosis.** The DDx of proteinuria vs. nephrotic syndrome is shown in Fig. 14-1.

Urinary Tract Infection (see Colorplate D, 9)

I. **Definition.** Acute or chronic infection of any portion of the urinary tract often resulting in dysuria, urgency, and frequency.

II. **Pathophysiology**

A. Usually due to ascending urinary tract infection by fecal-perineal flora. Since female urethra is shorter, UTI generally more common in females than males (except for cases of congenital anomalies and prostatism). Instrumentation of urethra increases risk.

B. Most common organism is *Escherichia coli*. Others include *Klebsiella, Proteus,* enterococci.

III. **Clinical manifestations and differential diagnosis**

A. UTI must be distinguished from other causes of dysuria, frequency, urgency, and lower abdominal pain. These disorders include genital infections, external bladder compression, prostatitis.

B. **Differentiating features of lower and upper UTI**

Features	Lower (cystitis)	Upper (pyelonephritis)
Signs and Sx	Dysuria, dark foul-smelling urine	H/A, chills, fever, vomiting, back pain, CVA tenderness.
Lab data	Bacteriuria, pyuria	Bacteriuria, proteinuria, pyuria, leukocytosis (with left-shift). Chronic UTI may result in anemia, uremia, acidosis, HBP.

Gonorrhea and Syphilis (see Colorplate D, 7)

I. **Definition.** Gonorrhea and syphilis are two common sexually transmitted diseases.

II. **Pathophysiology**

A. **Gonorrhea.** Over 3,000,000 untreated cases in U.S.; caused by *Neisseria gonorrhoeae*, a gram-negative, kidney-shaped diplococcus usually found intracellularly (especially in PMNs) on Gram stain.

B. **Syphilis.** Over 400,000 untreated cases in U.S.; caused by *Treponema pallidum*, a spirochete 0.25 μ wide and 5–20 μ long. *T. pallidum* often invades the CNS and aorta, leading to the symptoms of meningovascular neurosyphilis, tabes dorsalis, aortic insufficiency, and aortic scarring.

III. **Clinical manifestations and differential diagnosis**

	Time from exposure to onset	Signs and Sx	Lab results
A. Gonorrhea	2–8 days	Dysuria, frequency, discharge. Often asymptomatic. Males often	Discharge smears show gram-negative diplococci. Selective medium

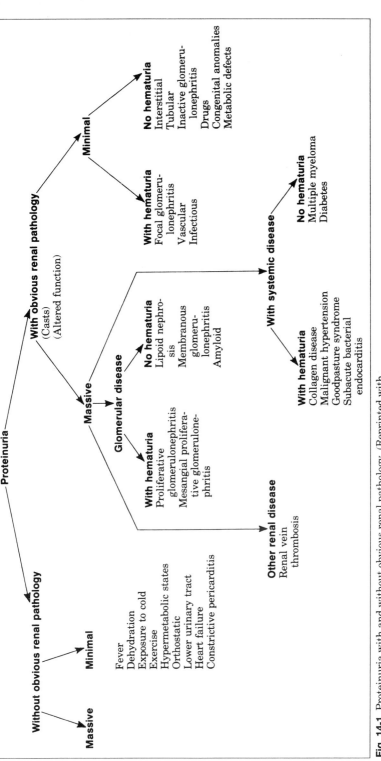

Fig. 14-1. Proteinuria with and without obvious renal pathology. (Reprinted with permission from J. W. Graef and T. E. Cone, Jr. [Eds.], *Manual of Pediatric Therapeutics* [2nd ed.]. Boston: Little, Brown, 1980.)

	Time from exposure to onset	Signs and Sx	Lab results
		present with urethritis, females with PID.	and high CO_2 necessary to culture organisms.
B. Primary syphilis	10–90 days (average 21)	Painless chancre, often in genital area. Nontender adenopathy in draining nodes.	Fluid from lesions contains *T. pallidum*; must use dark field or immunofluorescence.
C. Secondary syphilis	6 weeks–6 months	Mucosal lesions, generalized rash consisting of lesions (condylomata latum). Generalized nontender adenopathy. Fever, hepatitis, arthritis, iritis, meningitis.	VDRL and FTA-ABS serologic tests almost always positive.
D. Tertiary syphilis	2–10 years	Charcot's arthropathy, infiltrative tumors (gummas) in liver, skin, bone. Aortic aneurysms with aortic insufficiency. Meningovascular involvement.	Often positive CSF serology.
		CNS Sx: degenerative changes, tabes dorsalis, paresthesias, dementia, etc. Argyll Robertson pupil and Romberg sign.	

15

Hematologic and Oncologic
Diseases

Bleeding Disorders

I. **Definition.** Disorders of any element of the hemostatic system that result in an increased tendency to bleed.

II. **Pathophysiology**

   A. **Platelets** have a 10-day circulating lifespan; young platelets generally are larger and denser. Platelets aggregate at vascular injury sites and form plugs prior to clotting.

   B. **Coagulation cascade** involves sequences of plasma protein activations in two pathways. The **intrinsic pathway** begins with activation of factor XII, while the **extrinsic pathway** begins with exposure of plasma to tissue factor, which subsequently complexes with factor VII. Both pathways result in the activation of factor X, which then activates prothrombin to thrombin. The final stages of coagulation involve the conversion of prothrombin to thrombin, which in turn activates fibrinogen to fibrin. Factor XIII then catalyzes the conversion of fibrin to stabilized fibrin.

III. **Clinical manifestations and differential diagnosis of common bleeding disorders**

Disease	Description and pathophysiology	Characteristic findings
A. Platelet disorders		
1. Immune thrombocytopenic purpura (ITP)	Platelet destruction often due to antiplatelet antibody; normal numbers of megakaryocytes.	Platelets < 50,000; petechiae; purpura.
2. Thrombotic thrombocytopenic purpura (TTP)	Unknown etiology; often accompanied by DIC-like picture.	Purpura; thrombocytopenia; renal and neurologic problems; hemolytic anemia.

The clinician should not be deluded into believing that a tumor's complete clinical disappearance, even when microscopically "verified," necessarily carries any implications regarding long-term local control. A tumor may contain tens of millions of cells and not be clinically or pathologically evident. In addition, the clinical assumption that rapidly *responsive* tumors are extremely *sensitive* to antineoplastic agents has led to inadequate treatment in many cases. Only the passage of an appropriate amount of time allows a physician to make reasonably accurate estimations regarding the likelihood of ultimate cure.

J. Robert Cassady, M.D.

The most important event in determining the success of cancer therapy is the initial management decision. *Treatment goals must be clearly defined.* If cure is the goal then bold steps may be taken, but if palliation is the goal then the treatment should be designed to relieve symptoms while producing as few as possible.

Samuel Hellman, M.D.

Disease	Description and pathophysiology	Characteristic findings
3. Toxin-related thrombocytopenia	**Common agents:** EtOH, quinidine, thiazide diuretics, heparin, methyldopa, radiation, sulfonamides; mechanisms include platelet destruction and marrow failure.	Often severe, sudden onset thrombocytopenia, which usually resolves after agent discontinued.
B. Inherited coagulation defects		
1. Classic hemophilia (type A)	X-linked recessive gene; functionally inactive factor VIII.	Episodic visceral CNS and soft-tissue bleeding; hematuria; hemarthroses; may lead to osteoporosis.
2. Von Willebrand's disease	Often autosomal dominant; decreased von Willebrand's factor (which functions in combination with factor VIII) results in decreased platelet adhesiveness.	Normal platelet count; GI hemorrhage; epistaxis; bruising.
C. Acquired coagulation defects		
1. Disseminated intravascular coagulation (DIC)	Inappropriate activation of coagulation cascade leading to consumption of fibrinogen and other factors; often secondary to infection, tumors, shock.	Increased fibrin-split products; microangiopathic hemolytic anemia; embolic and thrombotic phenomena.
2. Vitamin K deficiency or malabsorption	Defective synthesis of factors II, VII, IX, X.	Prolonged PT; same clinical picture as that for hemophilia.
3. Liver failure	Often secondary to EtOH.	Decreased albumin; often decreased platelets secondary to hypersplenism; may be same clinical picture as that for hemophilia.

Anemia

I. **Definition.** Subnormal concentration of circulating erythrocytes or hemoglobin; roughly, Hct < 36%, Hgb < 12 gm/100 ml.

II. **Clinical manifestations and differential diagnosis of major types of anemia**

Type	Pathophysiology	Clinical picture	Lab abnormalities
A. Fe^{2+} deficiency	Depletion of iron stores (often due to blood loss) causing defective hemoglobin production.	Pallor; fatigue; brittle nails; tachycardia; pica. Increase in anginal Sx.	Hypochromic microcytic smear; ↓ serum ferritin; absent or low serum and marrow iron; ↑ TIBC; platelets and reticulocytes ↑ or normal.

Type	Pathophysiology	Clinical picture	Lab abnormalities
B. Megaloblastic anemia	Faulty erythropoiesis due to ↓ nucleic acid synthesis; often secondary to deficiency of B_{12} or gastric intrinsic factor (*pernicious anemia*) or to folic acid deficiency.	Anorexia; sore tongue; pallor; peripheral neuropathy; psychosis; gait disturbance.	Pancytopenia; hypersegmented PMNs; oval macrocytosis; megaloblastic marrow; low serum B_{12} or folate.
C. Hemolytic anemias: congenital			
1. Hereditary spherocytosis	Autosomal dominant defect in RBC spectrin causing ↑ permeability to Na^+.	Anemia; splenomegaly; jaundice; gallstones; malaise.	↑ Osmotic fragility of RBCs; spherocytes; ↑ reticulocytes.
2. Hereditary nonspherocytic hemolytic anemias	Intrinsic RBC defects involving Embden-Meyerhof pathway (pyruvate kinase deficiency) and hexose monophosphate shunt (glucose-6-phosphate dehydrogenase deficiency).	Anemia; jaundice.	Abnormal G6PD or pyruvate kinase assay; polychromatophilia; poikilocytosis; ↑ reticulocytes.
3. Hemoglobinopathies (sickle cell diseases, thalassemias)	**Sickle cell:** Valine replaces glutamate in position 6 of beta chain. **Thalassemias:** Unbalanced alpha- or beta-globin chain synthesis.	**Sickle cell:** anemia; episodic crises with fever; pains; jaundice; sickled cells; poikilocytes; ↑ reticulocytes. **Thalassemia:** Anemia, hepatosplenomegaly, facial bossing.	Definitive Dx by sickle test and Hgb electrophoresis; sickle smear shows sickled cells, fragmented forms, stomatocytes. **Thalassemia:** Hypochromic microcytosis, poikilocytes, target cells.
D. Hemolytic anemias: acquired			
1. Paroxysmal nocturnal hemoglobinuria	RBC membrane defect resulting in complement-mediated nocturnal hemolysis.	Weakness; jaundice; chills; fever; pain; hemoglobinuria; recurrent infections; thromboses; aplastic crises.	Abnormal Ham test; polychromatophilia.

Type	Pathophysiology	Clinical picture	Lab abnormalities
E. Aplastic anemias	Defective hematopoiesis due to congenital defects (Fanconi's), drug (chloramphenicol) reactions, infections, irradiation, neoplasms, idiopathic processes.	Pallor; bleeding; lassitude.	Fatty hypocellular marrow; normochromic normocytic anemia; pancytopenia.

Leukemias

I. **Definition:** A heterogeneous group of white blood cell malignancies resulting in either a rapidly progressive accumulation of immature leukocytes (**acute leukemias**) or a somewhat more indolent overgrowth by relatively mature leukocytes (**chronic leukemias**).

II. **Pathophysiology**

A. Cytokinetics of leukemic cells involve slow, incomplete, or defective maturation; longer than average cell survival time; lack of control by normal myelopoietic feedback systems.

B. **Etiology** unknown. Major speculations include viral agents, defective DNA repair, oncogenes.

III. **Clinical manifestations and differential diagnosis**

A. **Acute leukemias**

Feature	Acute lymphocytic (ALL)	Acute nonlymphocytic (AnLL or AML)
1. Epidemiology	Major childhood malignancy; rare in adults.	Uncommon; possible etiologic factors include radiation, chemicals, viruses.
2. Clinical manifestations	Infection; weakness; bleeding; anemia; lymphadenopathy.	Similar to ALL.
3. Physical exam	Pallor; fever; ecchymoses; adenopathy; hepatosplenomegaly.	Similar to ALL but less adenopathy and organomegaly.
4. Lab findings	↑ WBC; ↑ lymphocytes (especially immature forms); anemia; ↓ platelets; ↑ uric acid.	Anemia; ↓ platelets; moderate ↑ WBC (usually myeloblasts); ↑ uric acid; abnormal LFTs.
5. Clinical notes	CNS prophylaxis crucial; CNS and testicle are "sanctuaries" for leukemic cells; most lymphoblasts are "null" cells; T cell ALL has worse prognosis than null cell ALL.	DIC, leukostasis, and intracranial bleeds are common complications; at least 30–50% of patients have chromosome abnormality in leukemic cells; 50% of patients have **Auer rods** in myeloblasts (pathognomonic); peroxidase ⊕ cytoplasmic granules often found in malignant cells.

B. Chronic Leukemias

Feature	Chronic lymphocytic (CLL)	Chronic nonlymphocytic (CML)
1. Epidemiology	Disease of old age (usually over age 60); highest prevalence of any leukemia.	2 : 1 male-female; disease of middle age.
2. Clinical manifestations	Fatigue; weight loss; anorexia; pallor; fever; splenomegaly; mean survival after clinical onset 7–8 years.	Similar to CLL; mean survival after diagnosis 3–4 years.
3. Physical exam	Pallor; tachycardia; hepatosplenomegaly.	Lymphadenopathy, hepatosplenomegaly.
4. Lab findings	Often extreme ↑ WBC (especially mature small lymphocytes).	↑ WBC; basophilia; mild anemia; 90% of patients have Philadelphia chromosome; usually low leukocyte alkaline phosphatase values.
5. Clinical notes	Malignant cell usually monoclonal B lymphocyte with defective IgG production; ↓ immune defense, so infection common; hemolytic anemia frequent complication.	Chronic disease usually lasts 2–5 years, followed by **blast crisis,** in which mature myelocytes are replaced by immature myeloblasts, promyelo-blasts, and/or lympho-blasts, with survival time of 6 months.

Colorectal Carcinoma

I. **Definition.** Colorectal Ca is the second (after lung cancer) most common cause of cancer deaths in the U.S. (51,000/yr). Male-female ratio is 1 : 1; peak incidence in patients over 60 years.

II. **Pathophysiology**

   A. 50% in rectum, 20% sigmoid, 16% cecum; usually adenocarcinoma.

   B. Adenomatous polyps may be premalignant precursor; sessile polyps have higher incidence of invasive malignant foci than pedunculated polyps.

   C. Risk factors include Hx of ulcerative colitis, familial polyposis, Gardner's syndrome, FHx of colonic cancer.

   D. Mucosal environment may be a critical factor; low-fiber diets and long bowel transit times may be risk factors.

III. **Clinical manifestations**

   A. Common presentations include change in bowel habits, abdominal pain, tenesmus, weight loss, fatigue, hemorrhoids, change in stool caliber.

   B. Important lab investigations include tests for occult stool blood, barium enema, low hematocrit. Carcinoembryonic antigen (CEA) may be elevated, especially in patients with metastases.

IV. Staging and prognosis

Classification

Dukes	Modified Astwood-Coller	Description	Percent 5-year survivals
A	A	Lesion limited to mucosa; nodes negative	80%
B	B$_1$	Extension of lesion through mucosa but still within bowel wall; nodes negative	70%
	B$_2$	Extension through the entire bowel wall (including serosa); nodes negative	60–65%
C	C$_1$	Lesion limited to bowel wall; nodes positive	35–45%
	C$_2$	Extension of lesion through entire bowel wall (including serosa); nodes positive	15–30%

Breast Cancer

I. **Definition.** Breast cancer is the most common malignant tumor found in nonsmoking American women; incidence is ~ 70 in 100,000 women.

II. **Pathophysiology**

   A. Histologically 75% are classified as ductal adenocarcinomas; other types include lobular, medullary, and colloid carcinomas.

   B. Risk factors include FHx, high-fat diets (↑ steroid precursors?), and high estriol-to-estrone + estrodiol ratio. Nulliparous and late first pregnancy women may be at increased risk. Unclear whether oral contraceptives are risk factors.

   C. Usual routes of metastasis

   1. Regional metastasis by way of axillary and internal mammary lymph node chains.

   2. Distant metastases (lymphatic and hematogenous) to bones, lungs, liver.

III. **Clinical manifestations**

   A. Common presentations. Painless breast mass, nipple discharge, erythema, dimpling of breast skin, axillary and supraclavicular adenopathy.

   B. Pertinent lab investigations. Mammography, CXR, bone scans, LFTs, CEA titer, biopsy (with estrogen receptor protein level analysis).

   C. Paget's disease. Nipple is crusted and eczematous due to malignant infiltration along nipple ducts from deep tumor.

IV. Differential diagnosis and staging

A. Breast carcinoma must be differentiated from benign breast masses: polycystic breast disease and adenofibromas. In contrast to malignancy, both benign conditions are well delineated and mobile, without signs of retraction. Mammography is often helpful. **Biopsy results are definitive.** Estrogen receptor protein helps predict therapeutic response.

B. Clinical stage vs. survival rate for breast Ca

Stage		Survival (%)	
		2 yr	**5 yr**
I	tumor < 2 cm	95%	82%
II	tumor 2–5 cm; regional nodes ⊕ or ⊖	89%	63%
III	tumor > 5 cm; or extensions to other structures; regional nodes ⊕ or ⊖	70%	42%
IV	distant metastases	22%	< 10%

Lung Cancer

I. Definition. Lung cancer represents 22% of cancer in American men, 6% of cancer in American women. Most common fatal cancer in U.S.

II. Pathophysiology

A. Lung Ca is classified histologically into four types:

1. Squamous or epidermoid (30–40%).

2. Adenocarcinoma (30–40%).

3. Small cell (oat cell) (20%).

4. Giant cell (5–15%).

B. Small cell cancer may be different from the other types since it may arise from neuroectodermal (APUD) cells. These cells contain neurosecretory granules and active aromatic amines, and may secrete a variety of bioactive polypeptides and amines. It is the most rapidly fatal of the cell types (5-year survival < 1%) if untreated.

C. Etiologic risk factors include cigarettes, asbestos, radiation, industrial chemicals (e.g., nickel, chromate), and perhaps high endogenous concentrations of aryl hydrocarbon hydroxylase in bronchial epithelium.

D. Adenocarcinoma most common pathologic type in nonsmoking women.

III. Clinical manifestations

A. Symptoms depend on location and extent of tumor: weight loss, cough, wheezing, hemoptysis, dyspnea, ↑ sputum production (positive cytology may be diagnostic) are common presentations for endobronchial tumor. Chest pain or pleural effusion suggests extension to pleura and chest wall. Vena cava obstruction and tracheal-esophageal symptoms common if tumor invades mediastinum.

B. Metastases (lymphatic and hematogenous spread) occur early, most often to bones, lymphoreticular system, CNS, liver, and skin.

C. Endocrine, neurologic, connective tissue, and cutaneous manifestations also common (paraneoplastic syndromes), especially with small cell carcinoma.

IV. Differential diagnosis. Most important DDx is between malignancy and benign processes (most commonly granulomas) that appear as coin lesions on chest x-ray. Important tests include comparison of current CXR with old films, sputum cytology, tuberculin and fungal skin tests, and fiberoptic bronchoscopy.

Feature	Bronchogenic carcinoma	Granuloma (tuberculosis, histoplasmosis, coccidiomycosis)
Epidemiology	Smoker over age 35	Any age; geographic background important
Constitutional and respiratory symptoms	Cough, hemoptysis, wheeze, weight loss	Often absent
CXR appearance of coin lesion	Stellate border, not calcified	Calcified, with sharp margins
	Lesion doubles in size in 37–465 days	Radiographically unchanged over 2-year period *or* grows more rapidly or slowly than carcinoma limits

Acquired Immune Deficiency Syndrome (AIDS)

I. Definition. A syndrome generally recognized since 1979, characterized by evidence of HTLV–3 (HIV) viral infection or evidence of unexplained deficits in cell-mediated immunity leading to unusual opportunistic infections or malignancies (see sec. **V.B.**).

II. Pathophysiology. HIV is found in blood, semen, and saliva of infected individuals. Immunodeficiency thought due to viral infection of T lymphocytes, especially T4 + ("helper") cells. This results in a decrease in total lymphocyte count as well as a decrease in ratio of T4 + helper to T8 + "suppressor" cells (normal ratio approximately 2 : 1; classic AIDS ratio less than 1 : 1).

III. Epidemiology. At present, more than 1,000,000 United States citizens show evidence of HIV infection but approximately 50,000 have full clinical syndrome. High risk groups include male homosexuals, IV drug users and their recent offspring, heavily transfused patients and hemophiliacs, and perhaps Haitians and central Africans.

IV. Presenting symptoms include:

A. Generalized lymphadenopathy.

B. Fatigue, fever, failure to thrive.

C. Diarrhea.

D. AIDS-associated malignancies.

E. Atypical infections (see sec. **V.B.**).

V. Major clinical sequella

A. May be asymptomatic for years in prodrome phase (AIDS-related complex [ARC]).

B. Full blown AIDS often involves:

   1. Candida or herpes mucosal infection.

   2. *Pneumocystis carinii* or atypical *mycobacterium* pneumonia.

   3. Cryptococcal meningitis.

   4. CMV encephalitis.

   5. Unusual malignancy such as Kaposi's sarcoma or lymphoma of the CNS.

VI. Treatment. There is currently no good treatment for AIDS. Opportunistic infections are treated on an ad hoc basis. Infections and malignancies often recur regularly. True AIDS is thought to be universally fatal.

16

Pulmonary Diseases

Asthma

I. **Definiton.** Syndrome of reversible airway hyperreactivity in response to a number of known stimuli (extrinsic asthma) or no identifiable stimulus (intrinsic asthma).

II. **Pathophysiology.** Mechanism of bronchospasm not fully defined; involves chemical mediators from bronchial mast cells, parasympathetic nervous system. Mast cell mediator formation inhibited by cyclic adenosine monophosphate (**cAMP**). Smooth muscle contractions, bronchial wall edema, thickened secretions all lead to diminished airway diameter.

III. **Clinical manifestations**

A. Findings associated with the two general classes of asthma, **extrinsic** and **intrinsic,** are compared below.

Class	Inciting agent	Age	Historical points	PE	Lab
Ex-trinsic	Pollen; animal dander	70% of asthmatics < 30 yr	Spring-fall hay fever; ± infantile eczema; FHx allergies	Urticaria; eczema; chest exam findings (see **C**)	↑ Circulating IgE; skin tests positive
Intrinsic	Upper respiratory infections; emotional factors; nonspecific irritants	70% of asthmatics > 30 yr	± H/O ↑ in winter; chronic cough; H/O respiratory infections; subset with salicylate intolerance	Rhinitis; nasal polyps; chest exam findings (see **C**)	Normal IgE levels; skin tests negative

B. **Other possible provocative factors** include salicylates, nonsteroidal antiinflammatory drugs, Isocyanate, exercise, and cold weather.

C. **PE**

1. Pulsus paradoxus (reflects large intrapleural pressure swings).

Many patients with lung disease have important occupational and environmental factors in their histories. It is important to obtain a detailed and chronological work history and environmental exposure record going back to school days, including summer jobs, hobbies, and pastimes. Latency and chronicity are the hallmarks of many occupationally related disorders of the respiratory system.

In thinking of **causes of dyspnea**, it is necessary not only to think of cardiac and respiratory system disease, but also of anemia, primary muscle disease, as well as simple inactivity.

Homayoun Kazemi, M.D.

    2. Sternocleidomastoid muscle retractions.

    3. Lungs: inspiratory-expiratory rhonchi, hyperinflated chest, prolonged expiratory phase, frank wheezing, obvious respiratory distress, cyanosis in severe cases.

D. Lab findings

    1. CBC. Eosinophilia; ↑ WBC may be associated with an inciting infection; most associated pneumonias are viral.

    2. Sputum. Eosinophilia; bronchial casts; possible aspergillosis; ± Curshmann's spirals; ± Charcot-Leyden crystals.

    3. CXR. Hyperinflation; pneumonia; atelectasis.

    4. ABGs. Variable; often ↓ PO_2; ↓ PCO_2 reflects hyperventilation (normal or ↑ PCO_2 may be sign of impending respiratory failure).

    5. PFTs. FEV_1 ↓ ↓; FVC ↓ ↓; RV ↑; TLC ↑ acutely; subtle similar abnormalities may persist chronically.

Chronic Obstructive Pulmonary Disease (COPD)

I. Definitions

    A. Chronic bronchitis is a clinical syndrome characterized by excessive tracheobronchial mucus secretion so as to produce cough with sputum production on most days for at least 3 months of the year, during 2 or more consecutive years.

    B. Emphysema is a morphologic diagnosis characterized histologically by distention of the air spaces distal to the terminal bronchiole with destruction of alveolar walls.

    COPD is thus **chronic airflow obstruction secondary to chronic bronchitis and/or emphysema.**

II. Pathophysiology

    A. Chronic bronchitis is characterized by hypertrophy and hyperplasia of submucosal mucus-producing glands in larger airways, and small airway changes such as goblet-cell hyperplasia, inflammatory reaction, and retained bronchial secretions. **Cigarette smoking** plays a central role in etiology of chronic bronchitis.

    B. Emphysema is subdivided into two main types: **panacinar** and **centrilobular.** Panacinar form shows uniform destruction of the acinus, tends to occur in dependent portions of the lung, and is more likely to lead to bullae formation. Centrilobular emphysema tends to leave alveoli at margin of acinus unaffected; it generally involves alveolar ducts and respiratory bronchioles in the center of the lobule. Clinically, emphysema is best diagnosed by spirometric tests (which correlate well with the pathologic changes that define the disease).

III. Clinical manifestations and differential diagnosis. COPD is rarely pure; more often it is a mixture of chronic bronchitis and emphysematous disease.

Features	Type A	Type B
A. Type	Emphysematous (pink puffer)	Chronic bronchitic (blue bloater)
B. Hx/Sx		
1. Dyspnea	Insidious onset; often becomes severe	Mild to severe
2. Cough	Follows dyspnea	Precedes dyspnea
3. Sputum	Scant; mucoid	Copious; purulent
4. Rest symptoms	Marked	Milder
5. Weight change	Often marked loss	Slight loss to moderate gain

Features	Type A	Type B
6. Bronchial infections	Less frequent	More frequent
7. Respiratory insufficiency episodes	At terminal course	Common and repeated
8. Age at diagnosis	± 60 yr	± 50 yr
C. PE findings		
1. Integument	No cyanosis or clubbing	Cyanosis; rarely, clubbing
2. Pulmonary	Hyperresonance; end-expiratory wheezing; lower ICS retractions; accessory muscle usage	No hyperresonance; often rhonchi with coarse and wet breath sounds; no lower ICS retraction; less accessory muscle usage
D. Pulmonary function studies		
1. Total lung capacity	Increased	Normal or slightly increased or decreased
2. Vital capacity	Decreased	Decreased
3. Residual volume	Greatly increased	Moderately increased
4. Elastic recoil	Markedly decreased	Normal
5. Inspiratory airway resistance	Normal to slightly increased	Markedly increased
6. Compliance (static)	Increased	Near normal
7. Compliance (dynamic)	Normal to slightly decreased	Markedly decreased
E. Lab findings		
1. Hematocrit	35–45%	40–55% (lower value may indicate superimposed infection with anemia)
2. $PaCO_2$	35–40 mm Hg	50–65 mm Hg
3. PaO_2	65–75 mm Hg	45–60 mm Hg
4. Diffusing capacity	Decreased	Normal to slightly decreased
5. Cardiac output	Often decreased	Usually normal
6. Chest x-ray	Hyperlucent, overinflated lung with flat diaphragms; small heart	Large heart; increased bronchovascular shadows in lower field; evidence of old inflammatory disease
F. Complications		
1. Pulmonary hypertension		
a. Rest	None to mild	Moderate to severe
b. Exercise	Moderate	Worsens
2. Cor pulmonale	Rare (terminal event)	Common
3. Infectious exacerbations	Less frequent	More common

Pulmonary Tuberculosis (see Colorplate D, 11)

I. **Definition.** A chronic, necrotizing, transmissible infection of the lungs caused by *Mycobacterium tuberculosis*.

II. **Pathophysiology**

A. Infection in Western societies almost always is by inhalation of aerosolized bacilli ("droplet nuclei") from coughing, sneezing, or speech. Tubercle bacilli multiply slowly (maximum of 1–2 cell divisions/day) and require high O_2 concentration.

B. Disease stages

1. **Primary TB.** Bacterial multiplication with asymptomatic spread to regional hilar nodes; leads to lymphohematogenous spread. Seeds widely, especially to the lung apices, kidneys, spine–long bones, brain, lymph nodes (organs with high oxygen concentrations). Reticuloendothelial system involved in clearance of bacilli.

2. **Post–primary TB.** Onset 3–6 weeks after infection; a specific population of T lymphocytes determines pathologic response and is responsible for tuberculin reaction and cellular immunity. Quiescent TB results from immunologically contained infection.

III. Clinical manifestations

A. Symptoms. Often asymptomatic (CXR discovery). Initial constitutional symptoms: anorexia, ↓ weight, fever, chills, fatigue, night sweats. Dyspnea, cough, sputum, hemoptysis, and pleuritic pain.

B. PE findings. There may be none. Possible associated findings are asymmetric respiratory excursion ± tracheal deviation, dullness to percussion, ↑ tactile fremitus over involved areas, rales (**posttussive** classically).

C. Lab findings

PPD	Negative TB with positive *Candida* or mumps control is highly sensitive in excluding active TB. A positive PPD is common in older populations. **Recent conversion** to a positive PPD is usually significant. Patients who have received **BCG vaccine** will be PPD positive.
Sputum	AFB stain positive in primary TB, although it is often difficult to find the organism microscopically.
CBC	Normochromic, normocytic anemia common (may be severe); WBC normal (diff may include 8–15% mononuclear cells).
U/A	Hematuria and pyuria may indicate renal involvement (**sterile pyuria** classically associated with TB). Albuminuria (secondary amyloidosis) may be seen in prolonged infections.
Chemistry	↓ Na (SIADH) ↓ Albumin (severe cases)

D. Chest x-ray. CXR is crucial to diagnosis. In primary TB it often reveals patchy infiltrates in lower lung fields and hilar adenopathy. In post–primary TB, patchy apical infiltrates, cavitation, fibronodular infiltrates, and fibrosis are common.

IV. Differential diagnosis

	Comments
A. Acute bacterial pneumonia	Sputum exam, response to antibiotics helpful in distinguishing from TB.
B. Neoplasm	High incidence of tuberculous changes in upper lobes of older men may make the DDx confusing; sputum cytology, bronchoscopy with brushings may help distinguish.
C. Sarcoidosis	Negative TB test; lymph node biopsy through mediastinoscopy may be necessary to distinguish.
D. Fungal disorder (especially histoplasmosis)	Histoplasmosis and TB may coexist; skin tests for fungus and cultures help make the Dx.
E. Cavitary lung abscess	Involves superior segments of lower lobes (most often due to aspiration); positive air-fluid level (rare in TB); no associated patchy infiltrate adjacent to cavity on CXR (common in TB).

Pulmonary Embolism

I. Definition. Impaction of thrombotic or other foreign matter in the pulmonary vascular bed.

II. Pathophysiology

    A. Between 80 and 90% are due to venous thrombi originating in the lower extremities; in postsurgical patients, pelvic vein or prostatic plexus thrombi may also lead to emboli.

    B. Predisposing factors include immobilization (including that of chronically ill medical patients), venous disease, prior cardiopulmonary disease, oral contraceptives, pregnancy, surgery, trauma, and carcinoma.

III. Clinical manifestations

    A. Symptoms. Anxiety, restlessness, diaphoresis, sudden onset of dyspnea, precordial or substernal pain, sudden cough or hemoptysis, syncope.

    B. PE findings

        1. General. Tachypnea, tachycardia, hypotension, cyanosis, fever.

        2. Pulmonary. Rales, ronchi, wheezes, pleural friction rub.

        3. CV. Distended neck veins, S_2 (P_2 component), pulmonary artery pulsation, S_4 (and/or S_3), systolic-diastolic murmurs. There may also be positive hepatojugular reflux, hepatomegaly, and evidence for severe right heart failure in patients with multiple chronic pulmonary embolization.

    C. Lab findings

        1. ECG. Normal in many patients. There may be transient, variable changes, including T wave inversion in V_1 to V_3, and acute cor pulmonale with "S1Q3T3" pattern, RBBB, RAD in 25% of patients. There may also be poor R wave progression as enlarged RV displaces LV posteriorly.

        2. CXR. Normal in 50% of patients. There may be also abrupt cut-off of vessel shadow and radiolucent area distal to the area of embolus (**Westermark's sign**). Atelectatic streaks and consolidated areas may be present, as may pleural effusion or unilateral elevation of diaphragm.

        3. ABGs. $\downarrow$ PaO_2 (on room air); $\downarrow$ PCO_2 (hyperventilation).

IV. Differential diagnosis. Note that the symptoms and signs of pulmonary embolism are **nonspecific**; it is a difficult diagnosis to make. Use the following parameters in considering the diagnosis:

    A. Clinical story (strong suspicion crucial).

    B. CXR.

    C. ABGs.

    D. Pleural effusion (PE is 1 of 4 causes of > 100,000 RBCs in a pleural effusion; the others are TB, malignancy, and trauma).

    E. Ventilation-perfusion isotope lung scan mismatches.

    F. Pulmonary arteriogram is the "gold standard" for diagnosis.

Common Pneumonias (see Colorplate D)

I. Definition. A group of microbial infections of pulmonary tissue that produce a spectrum of clinical responses characterized by varying degrees of cough, fever, and pulmonary symptoms.

II. Clinical manifestations and differential diagnosis. Some of the most common bacterial, viral, and fungal pneumonias are compared below.

Type	Clinical manifestations	CXR	DDx and comments
A. Bacterial pneumonias			
1. *Streptococcus pneumoniae* (pneumococcus) (see Colorplate D, 6)	H/O preceding upper respiratory infection, classically with single, violent shaking chill at onset; fever ≥ 102° F; sustained pleuritic chest pain often present with cough, chills; "rust" or blood-stained sputum may be present; associated herpes labialis (cold sore).	Lobar consolidation (although may give any other pattern).	Patient appears seriously ill. Check for egophony and friction rubs over areas of consolidation. Abdominal distention frequently present. Gram stain is better diagnostically than culture, which often fails to grow organism. Positive blood culture in 20–25% of patients allows definitive diagnosis.
2. *Klebsiella pneumoniae* (Friedländer's pneumonia) (see Colorplate D, 10)	Sudden onset of symptoms with fever ≥ 102° F, chills, cough, and thick, bloody ("tenacious") sputum.	Variable; upper lobe common; central cavitation and abscess formation may be seen.	Alcoholics especially predisposed, but also seen in diabetics, COPD patients.
3. *Staphylococcus aureus* (see Colorplate D, 2)	Fever > 102° F, chills, pleuritic pain, cough (may be nonproductive); thick, purulent, blood-streaked sputum (creamy, salmon, or red-yellow in color).	Bronchopneumonic pattern (often bilateral) seen; cavitation and abscesses common.	Necrotizing infection with high mortality rate. Higher incidence in infants, children with cystic fibrosis, postinfluenza in adults; also in debilitated populations, IV drug users. May arise from hematogenous spread, in which case PE signs are less prominent; infected skin site (portal of entry) often identifiable.
B. Mycoplasma pneumonias (*Mycoplasma pneumoniae*)	Nonspecific constitutional symptoms are of insidious onset with fever > 101° F, nonproductive persistent cough with scant mucoid sputum.	Interstitial pneumonia, usually unilateral; usually seen in lower lobes with ± small pleural effusions; radiologic findings often far more severe than clinical manifestations.	5–30 yr age group. Cough is dominant symptom; mild or absent cough makes the diagnosis suspect. PE findings may be minimal (rales, cough, but little else). Positive complement fixation

Type	Clinical manifestations	CXR	DDx and comments
			tests in 75–80% of patients. **Cold agglutinins** help make the diagnosis.
C. Viral pneumonias (Influenza)	Fever up to 105° F with hacking cough; sputum often blood-tinged.	Interstitial pattern seen (diffuse, generalized, infiltrate); hazy, reticular densities or discreet nodules and migratory consolidated areas may be present.	Patients appear less ill than those with bacterial pneumonias. Chest pain is rare, and pulmonary auscultatory findings may be minimal or absent; respiratory insufficiency may be out of proportion to CXR.
D. Fungal pneumonias			
1. *Histoplasma capsulatum*	Fever present; minimal or absent sputum with nonproductive cough; chills rare.	Lower lobes favored with generalized nodular and linear infiltrates; uni- or bilateral adenopathy may be present.	H/O contact with bird droppings may be present. Infants and older patients are predisposed. May be complicated by bacterial pneumonia.
2. *Coccidioides*	Often asymptomatic or flulike, with fever, night sweats, weight loss, rash; chills common.	Same as above.	Culture-serology necessary for diagnosis. Wide range of pulmonary syndromes are possible. May be associated with erythema nodosum. Southwestern U.S. distribution. Skin test and serologic test are helpful for Dx.

Thyrotoxicosis (Hyperthyroidism)

I. Definition. Clinical syndrome resulting from excess thyroid hormone.

II. Etiologies

	Pathophysiology
A. Grave's disease (usually autoimmune)	TSH-like immunoglobulins stimulate ↑ thyroid hormone
B. Toxic multinodular goiter	Multiple autonomous areas of thyroid tissue lead to ↑ thyroid hormone production
C. Toxic adenoma	Overproduction of thyroid hormone by a single "hot" nodule

D. Other less common causes include iatrogenic etiologies, thyroiditis-associated disorders, struma ovarii, TSH-like substance production by tumors, trophoblastic tumors, thyroid carcinoma, exogenous thyroid hormone.

III. Clinical manifestations. The protean clinical findings in thyrotoxicosis are outlined below by organ system.

Organ system	Symptoms	PE findings
A. Constitutional	Fatigue; hyperactivity; insomnia; heat intolerance; ↑ appetite; weight loss	Hyperkinetism; tremulousness
B. Vital signs		Tachycardia; tachypnea; pyrexia; wide pulse pressure
C. Integument	Sweating; ↑ hair growth; pruritus; occasional urticaria	Warm, moist, fine hair; pretibial myxedema*; onycholysis; hyperpigmentation
D. Eyes*	Complaints of visual disturbance	Lid lag, stare, proptosis*, inflammation, ophthalmoplegia (upward gaze affected first), chemosis, periorbital edema
E. Neck	Complaints of neck mass	Goiter, lymphadenopathy
F. CV	Palpitations; dyspnea	Hyperdynamic precordium; arrhythmias (new onset of atrial fibrillation or tachycardia)

*Specifically characteristic of Graves' disease.

In differential diagnosis of hypercalcemia, chronicity of the illness is a key clinical issue. Median survival after onset of hypercalcemia in tumor-related humoral hypercalcemia is less than 6 months; evidence of chronicity (e.g., kidney stones or hypercalcemia of many months duration) favors hyperparathyroidism or sarcoidosis.

John T. Potts, Jr., M.D.

	Organ system	**Symptoms**	**PE findings**
G.	GI	Increasing frequency of bowel movements; diarrhea	Active bowel sounds; splenomegaly*
H.	GU/GYN	Nocturia, oligomenorrhea	
I.	Neuromuscular	Muscle weakness; tremor	Proximal muscle weakness; tremor; brisk deep tendon reflexes
J.	Psychological	Emotional lability; nervousness	

Hypercalcemia

I. **Definition.** An elevation of ionized calcium in serum.

II. **Pathophysiology.** The two most important regulators of calcium metabolism are **parathyroid hormone (PTH)** and the renal metabolite of vitamin D, **1,25(OH)$_2$ vitamin D.**

$$\begin{array}{c} \nearrow \quad \uparrow \text{ renal phosphorus excretion} \\ \text{PTH} \rightarrow \quad \uparrow \text{ 1,25(OH)}_2\text{D} \quad \text{production} \rightarrow \uparrow \text{intestinal Ca}^{2+} \\ \searrow \quad \text{mobilization} \\ \downarrow \\ \uparrow \text{ bone mobilization of Ca}^{2+} \text{ [probably synergistic with 1,25(OH)}_2\text{D]} \end{array}$$

III. **Etiology.** The two most common causes are **malignancy** and **primary hyperparathyroidism.** Malignancy is the most frequent cause in a hospital population while primary hyperparathyroidism is the most frequent cause in the general population.

A. Common malignancies	**Pathophysiology of hypercalcemia**
1. Multiple myeloma	Osteoclastic activating factor (OAF) production
2. Bone metastases (e.g., breast Ca)	Direct bone invasion, but ↑ calcium probably due to local mediator production (e.g., prostaglandins)
3. Squamous lung Ca, renal cell Ca	Ectopic PTH-like substance produced ("pseudohyperparathyroidism")
B. Primary hyperparathyroidism	Autonomous PTH production causing ↑ calcium (see **II**).

C. **Other less common causes** include sarcoidosis, vitamin D intoxication, thyrotoxicosis, milk-alkali syndrome, adrenal insufficiency, immobilization, vitamin A intoxication, and pheochromocytoma.

IV. **Clinical features**

A. **Symptoms** are generally related to neurologic and neuromuscular function.

Somnolence, apathy, memory loss, mental disturbances (severity proportional to degree of hypercalcemia), irritability, stupor-coma (c/w acute, pronounced hypercalcemia), and proximal muscle weakness are characteristic. Symptoms tend to be variable and nonspecific.

B. **PE findings** are rarely helpful for diagnosis of hypercalcemia. Some of those associated are band keratopathy, ↑ blood pressure, hypotonia, and ↓ deep tendon reflexes.

*Specifically characteristic of Graves' disease.

C. ECG shows ↓ Q-T interval, atrial arrhythmias, various AV blocks.

D. X-ray indicates soft tissue calcification.

E. Chemistry tests show elevated calcium. Calcium levels must be evaluated after **correction** of the measured level for the amount of **serum albumin** present. Since albumin binds calcium, the effective calcium level (ionized calcium) is related to the albumin concentration. Thus, for every 1.0-mg decrease in albumin, a 0.8-mEq decrease in serum calcium can be expected, and the corrected value is obtained by **adding** 0.8 mg/100 ml to the measured value for each 1.0-mg decrement in albumin. The converse is true for hyperalbuminemia. Two examples of how to calculate the "effective" calcium level follow.

Serum calcium	Albumin	Corrected (actual) serum calcium
7.5 mg/100 ml	2.0 mg/100 ml (decreased 2 mg)	9.1 mg/100 ml
11.0 mg/100 ml	5.0 mg/ 100 ml (increased 1 mg)	10.2 mg/100 ml

Hypercortisolism (Cushing's Syndrome)

I. **Definition.** Clinical and metabolic disease caused by glucocorticoid excess. **Cushing's disease** refers specifically to hyperfunction of hypothalamus and pituitary resulting in ↑ cortisol (see below).

II. **Etiologies.** Three types of endogenous hypercortisolism plus exogenous administration are the main causes.

    A. Hypothalamic-pituitary hyperfunction **(Cushing's disease).**

    B. Ectopic ACTH syndrome (causing **bilateral adrenal hyperplasia**).

    C. Unilateral autonomous adrenal hypersecretion (**adrenal adenoma** or carcinoma).

    D. Iatrogenic excess of any of several glucocorticoids.

III. **Clinical manifestations**

Symptom (approximate frequency)	Pathophysiology	Clinical points
Impaired glucose tolerance (94%)	Gluconeogenic effect of cortisol.	Most patients do not have clinical diabetes, only an abnormal glucose tolerance test.
Central (truncal) obesity (88%)	↑ Lipid mobilization, redistribution of adipose stores.	Extremities remain slender.
Hypertension (82%)	Accompanying mineralocorticoid activity.	Seen especially in ectopic ACTH syndrome; K$^+$ wasting.
Oligomenorrhea (72%)	Androgen excess.	↓ Fertility; virilism (hirsutism).
Osteoporosis (58%)	Antagonism of 1,25(OH)$_2$ vitamin D and inhibition of bone cell activation.	Secondary hyperparathyroidism; osteopenia on x-ray ("codfish" vertebrae).
Purpura and striae (42%)	Catabolic effects of cortisol.	Fragility of skin; ecchymoses.
Muscle atrophy-weakness (36%)	Catabolic effects of cortisol.	More severe cases; weakness may be extreme.

Strong clinical suspicion (heightened by presence of *several* of the above common clinical manifestations) is important for diagnosis.

IV. Lab work-up. Measurement of **morning plasma cortisol** or **urinary 17-OHCS**.

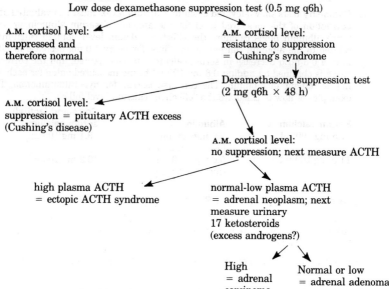

If elevated:
Low dose dexamethasone suppression test (0.5 mg q6h)

A.M. cortisol level:
suppressed and
therefore normal

A.M. cortisol level:
resistance to suppression
= Cushing's syndrome

Dexamethasone suppression test
(2 mg q6h × 48 h)

A.M. cortisol level:
suppression = pituitary ACTH excess
(Cushing's disease)

A.M. cortisol level:
no suppression; next measure ACTH

high plasma ACTH
= ectopic ACTH syndrome

normal-low plasma ACTH
= adrenal neoplasm; next
measure urinary
17 ketosteroids
(excess androgens?)

High
= adrenal
carcinoma

Normal or low
= adrenal adenoma

Diabetes Mellitus

I. Definition. Group of metabolic diseases resulting from absolute or relative insulin deficit; characterized by hyperglycemia and frequent ketosis.

II. Classification. Insulin-dependent and **insulin-independent** groups of diabetics may be identified. These two types of DM are compared in the table below.

		Insulin dependent	Insulin independent
A. Pathophysiology	**1.** Synonyms	"Brittle"; "ketosis-prone"; "juvenile-onset" DM (JODM).	"Maturity-onset," "late-onset," "non–insulin-dependent," or "adult-onset" DM (AODM); AODM seen in youths is sometimes called "maturity-onset diabetes of youth" (MODY).
	2. Usual pathophysiology	Decreased or absent insulin production from pancreatic cells.	Decreased or defective insulin receptors on target cells.
	3. Serum insulin levels	Decreased	Usually increased or normal
	4. Predisposing factors	Idiopathic (viral, autoimmune, genetic factors all probably important).	H/O obesity and FHx of DM. Seen also in pregnancy (gestational diabetes).
	5. Frequency	10–12% of cases.	80–85% of cases.
B. Clinical manifestations	**1.** Historical clues	< 30 yr at onset; inattentiveness in school, excessive craving for sweets, and increased ir-	Prior reactive hypoglycemia; H/O recurrent soft tissue or mycotic infections; females may have

B. Clinical manifestations	**Insulin dependent**	**Insulin independent**
1. Historical clues (continued)	ritability may all be early signs.	children born > 9 lb at birth.
2. Symptoms	Usually severe and progressive with anergic lassitude, weight loss, polyuria, polydipsia, polyphagia; blurred vision, leg cramps, mild to severe vomiting, and dehydration may appear if ketosis unattended.	Mild, often asymptomatic, on presentation, but then blurred vision, polyuria, polyphagia, polydipsia, if not treated; females may present with vaginitis; may be discovered during routine blood chemistries or urinalysis.

III. Chemical diagnosis. Increased fasting blood sugar (FBS) > 150 mg/dl; abnormal postprandial BS (if FBS normal); abnormal glucose tolerance test (GTT). Hemoglobin A_1C level is correlated with the degree of long-standing hyperglycemia and may be usual in monitoring the efficacy of long-term therapy in treated diabetics.

Musculoskeletal Diseases

Rheumatoid Arthritis

I. **Definition.** A chronic systemic disease characterized by inflammation of synovial membranes with resultant cartilage and joint destruction.

II. **Pathophysiology**

   A. **Etiology unknown** (autoimmune?); 3 : 1 female-male predominance. Risk factors include family history and HLA DW4.

   B. **Typical pathology** involves inflammation of the synovial membrane followed by hypertrophy and proliferation of the synovial membrane–lining cells (pannus tissue), which erode into the soft tissues of the joint. Microscopic findings include the **rheumatoid nodule,** a focus of central necrosis surrounded by a palisade of connective tissue cells and granulation tissue.

III. **Clinical manifestations. Onset** often insidious; may begin with small joints. **Prodromal Sx** include fever, malaise, weight loss, morning stiffness, lymphadenopathy. **Joint Sx** usually symmetric and include pain, swelling, stiffness, muscular weakness; in fingers, PIP and MCP joints usually involved, DIP relatively spared. As disease progresses, joint deformities develop, including ulnar deviation, hyperextension of PIP joints with flexion of the DIP joint ("swan-neck deformity"), and PIP flexion with DIP hyperextension ("boutonniere deformity").

IV. **Differential diagnosis of common joint diseases**

	RA	DJD	Gout
Important clinical differences	Morning stiffness	Lower extremities often involved	FHx

Assessment of the orthopaedic patient requires the same attention to historical detail and physical examination skills as in other disciplines but includes another feature: anatomical perception of the lesion and its effect on adjacent structures and function of the part. It is as patently inadequate to define an abnormal gait pattern as a "limp" as to describe a patient with aortic and mitral valvular lesions as having "heart disease." One must observe the patient closely; consider the anatomy of the affected part; the normal functional components of the support and movement activities of the site (and adjacent sites); analyze the pain pattern; and carefully record the aberrations seen in range of motion (active and passive), local structure, and complex activities (such as gait or prehension). Study of the x-ray is an integral part of the evaluation of the orthopaedic patient; it requires not only an appreciation of the normal anatomy but three-dimensional analysis of a two-dimensional radiograph. It is frequently the third dimension, rotational alteration, which is the clue to the value of the abnormality, be it genetic, traumatic, degenerative, inflammatory, metabolic, or neoplastic.

Henry J. Mankin, M.D.

Chronic low back pain in young men does not only indicate intervertebral disc disease. When the pain radiates down *both* buttocks, think of inflammatory disease such as ankylosing spondylitis. We still encounter such individuals who have gone through the diagnostic system with a myelogram, physical examination, and history in that order.

S. M. Krane, M.D.

	RA	DJD	Gout
Important clinical differences (continued)	Symmetric peripheral joint involvement	Relieved by rest	Acute onset, single joint affected
	Pain often migratory	Rare MCP and wrist involvement	Tophi
	Subcutaneous nodules	No constitutional manifestations	Urate crystals in synovial fluid
	Constitutional manifestations		Rare before puberty
	Absence of DIP involvement		Rare after menopause
	TM joint involvement	TMs rarely involved	Can be drug induced
X-ray	Periarticular osteoporosis	Narrowed joint space	Punched-out areas in bone due to radiolucent tophi
	Juxtaarticular erosions	Increased subchondral bone density	
	Subluxation of upper cervical spine common	Osteophytes	
		Subchondral crypts	
Lab	85% have positive rheumatoid factor (usually IgM reactive against IgG)	Lab values often normal	↑ ESR
			(Often ↑ uric acid in serum)
	Sometimes ⊕ANA test and usually ↑ ESR		
	Moderate anemia		

Degenerative Joint Disease

I. **Definition.** A chronic, progressive noninflammatory osteoarthropathy primarily involving the articular cartilage.

II. **Pathophysiology**

    A. **Primary DJD** affects DIP joints **(Heberden's nodes)** and PIP joints **(Bouchard's nodes)** as well as joints of thumb, hip, knee, cervical-lumbar spine. Etiology unknown; female predominance after age 45.

    B. **Secondary DJD** usually follows joint trauma; may affect any joint.

    C. **Classic DJD** pathology involves erosion of articular cartilage, bone spur formation (osteophytes), synovial hypertrophy with minimal inflammation.

III. **Clinical manifestations.** Onset usually insidious, with stiffness, pain, crepitus. Sx precipitated by activity and relieved by rest. Systemic involvement minimal. Entire disease may be asymptomatic.

IV. **Differential diagnosis.** See Rheumatoid Arthritis, sec. **IV.**

Systemic Lupus Erythematosus

I. **Definition.** An inflammatory autoimmune disease characterized by multiple organ involvement, joint symptoms, rash, and ⊕ANA test.

II. **Pathophysiology**

A. **Prevalence** approximately 1 in 2,000 persons; 8 : 1 female-male ratio; significant twin concordance.

B. **Etiology unknown**; some evidence for defective suppressor T cells allowing overactive B cells to produce autoantibodies. Viral infection may contribute to disease induction in susceptible hosts.

III. **Clinical manifestations**

A. **Systemic findings.** Fever, chills, malaise.

B. **Organ system findings.** Polyarthropathy, "cytoid bodies" in ocular fundus, pneumonitis, pericarditis, abdominal pain, hepatosplenomegaly, lymphadenopathy, lupus nephritis, CNS disturbances.

C. **Lab findings.** Normochromic, normocytic anemia; leukopenia; thrombocytopenia; ↑ ESR; false ⊕ serologic test for syphilis. Immunologic abnormalities include ↑ serum globulin, ⊕ Coombs test, ↓ serum complement, ⊕LE cells, autoantibodies to nucleic acids and ribonucleoprotein (**A**nti**N**uclear **A**ntibodies).

IV. **Differential diagnosis.** SLE must be distinguished from discoid lupus (skin rash without systemic disease), RA, and drug-induced lupus syndrome (hydralazine, Dilantin, procainamide). DDx often difficult and based on clinical picture and organ involvement.

19 Neurologic Diseases

Seizure Disorders (Epilepsy)

I. **Definition.** A group of disorders characterized by paroxysmal transitory changes in mental status and motor activity.

II. **Pathophysiology**

    A. Initial events in seizure cycle unclear. A group of neurons begins to fire synchronously, often recruiting neighboring groups. Seizures may be precipitated by drugs, hypoxia, hypoglycemia, and sensory stimulation.

    B. There are two general types of seizures:

        1. Focal seizures, which arise from discrete foci and may be due to local conditions (e.g., tumor, trauma).

        2. Generalized seizures, which are usually idiopathic or toxic-metabolic.

III. **Clinical manifestations and differential diagnosis.** The most important diagnostic and therapeutic issue to determine is the exact type of seizure. Many patients experience more than one type.

Seizure type	Characteristic findings
A. Focal	
1. Motor	Premonitory aura preceding focal convulsion; consciousness often retained; in Jacksonian epilepsy, there is a characteristic "March" of motor events as recruitment occurs.
2. Sensory	Flashing lights; tingling numbness; EEG often shows discharge in parietal and occipital lobes.
3. Temporal lobe	Automisms; patterned movements; emotional distress; hallucinations; dizziness; autonomic disorders.
B. Generalized	
1. Grand mal (tonic-clonic)	Tonic-clonic convulsions; loss of bowel-bladder control → flaccid coma → postictal confusion; no aura or focality.
2. Petit mal (absence)	Brief blank spells; myoclonic jerks; akinetic seizures; EEG shows 3 per second spike and wave morphology; common in children.

Often the cause of a *blackout* is apparent from what happens afterwards, more than from any premonitory symptoms. Patients who faint usually wake up immediately, and if in a crowd, find themselves surrounded by people staring down at them or attempting to help. Recovery of full awareness is rapid. This is true whether the syncope is on a vasovagal basis, or because of arrhythmia or bradycardia. On the other hand, a patient who had a seizure usually awakens in the ambulance or in the hospital, has a more gradual return of full consciousness, and often has muscle soreness and evidence of trauma to cheek or tongue. The patient who had a subarachnoid hemorrhage may awaken incompletely, and enter a state of combative confusion or stupor. This state may suggest that he has a postictal confusional state of alcohol intoxication when, in fact, it is a reflection of the blood in the subarachnoid space.

David M. Dawson, M.D.

Coma

I. Definition. A state of unconsciousness from which the patient cannot be aroused.

II. Pathophysiology

   A. Intracranial etiologies include trauma, vascular disease, tumors, CNS infections, seizure disorders, increased intracranial pressure.

   B. Extracranial etiologies include shock (including post-MI), metabolic disorders (hypoglycemia, uremia, hepatic disturbances, acidosis, electrolyte disturbances), drug effects, systemic trauma (hyperthermia, hypothermia, electric shock, anaphylaxis).

III. Clinical manifestations

   A. PE of patient in coma should include vital signs, pain responses, careful inspection (note especially **Battle's sign**, the discoloration of skin behind ear associated with skull fractures), pupillary and respiratory patterns, passive motion and "limb drop" maneuvers to search for hemiparesis, decerebrate or decorticate rigidity, nuchal rigidity, "doll's head" maneuver, ice water caloric response.

   B. Essential lab tests on comatose patients include CBC, U/A, ABG, ECG, electrolytes, blood alcohol and toxicology levels, liver and kidney function tests, glucose levels, PT, PTT. If indicated, LP and CT scan are performed.

IV. Differential diagnosis. Principal question is etiology of coma. A useful mnemonic to remember is **AEIOU TIPS** [15]:

Alcoholism
Encephalopathy
Insulin excess or deficiency
Opiates and other drugs
Uremia and metabolic disorders
Trauma
Infection
Psychiatric disorders
Syncope

Cerebrovascular Disorders (Stroke and Transient Ischemic Attack)

I. Definition. Acute derangement in neurologic function due to inadequate cerebral circulation. A transient ischemic attack (TIA) is any acute neurologic impairment that clears within 24 hours.

II. Pathophysiology. The three basic disease processes are:

   A. Thrombosis. Artheromatous thrombosis often involves large arteries, especially the carotid, vertebral, and basilar. **Hypertensive** thrombosis often affects the small arteries within the brain itself.

   B. Embolism. Often arises from the heart or calcific atherosclerotic plaques. Although emboli often occur in showers, they may affect individual cortical arteries, causing isolated cortical defects that appear and resolve suddenly.

   C. Hemorrhage. Often occurs secondary to trauma, rupture of congenital aneurysms, arteriovenous malformations, intracranial hypertensive ruptures.

III. Clinical manifestations. Premonitory signs may include H/A, dizziness, confusion. Sx of actual disorders depend on exactly which structures are affected. Classic TIA sign is "shade coming down over one eye" **(amaurosis fugax).** Strokes may be associated with vomiting, convulsions, fever, nuchal rigidity, changed mental status.

IV. Differential diagnosis. Common signs and Sx associated with occlusion of particular arteries follow:

Artery affected	Findings
Middle cerebral artery (MCA)	Contralateral hemiparesis (arm and face > leg); numbness; homonymous hemianopsia; aphasias; apraxia.
Anterior cerebral artery	Contralateral hemiplegia (maximal in the leg); grasp and suck reflexes; incontinence.
Posterior cerebral artery	Contralateral hemisensory loss; hemianopsia; visual defects; memory deficits.
Internal carotid artery	Variable; may be silent or may be similar to MCA stroke with profound changes in mental status. Upper extremity Sx are common.
Vertebrobasilar artery	May overlap with PCA stroke, with brainstem and/or cerebellar signs; ipsilateral cranial nerve problems; contralateral or bilateral motor, sensory, cerebellar signs; staggering gait; ataxia; dysphagia; confusion.

See Appendix A, Fig. A-1 for diagram of Circle of Willis.

Meningitis (see Colorplate D, 8)

I. **Definition.** Inflammation of the meninges of the brain or spinal cord, most often due to pneumococcus, *Neisseria meningitidis, Haemophilus influenzae,* mumps virus, or enteroviruses.

II. **Pathophysiology**

   A. Most common in children, elderly, and others with ↓ immunity.

   B. Entry may be through surgical or traumatic wound or through inhaled droplets. Gram-positive meningitis may follow an infection of the lungs, middle ear, or sinuses.

   C. Infection in subarachnoid space → inflammatory reaction in pia, arachnoid, and CSF → accumulation of pus or toxin → damage to nerve roots, choroid plexuses, microvasculature, and interference with CSF flow leading to hydrocephalus.

III. **Clinical manifestations.** There may be evidence of systemic infection: chills, fever, ↑ WBC, and lethargy. Further signs of meningitis include headache, vomiting, confusion, nuchal rigidity, convulsions, **Kernig's sign** (passive resistance to knee extension from flexed-thigh position), and **Brudzinski's sign** (neck flexion resulting in involuntary knee flexion in supine patient). Meningococcal meningitis is often associated with petechial mucous membrane and skin rashes.

IV. **Differential diagnosis on basis of CSF fluid (see Colorplate D)**

Disease type	CSF cell count	Predominant cell type in CSF	Glucose (mg/100 ml)	Protein (mg/100 ml)
Normal	< 5	Mononuclear	Two-thirds serum level or ~ 75	< 40
Bacterial meningitis	10–100,000	PMN	5–50	100–1,000
Viral Early phase	50–500	PMN	40–75	50–100
Late phase	20–200	Mononuclear	Normal	< 100

Disease type	CSF cell count	Predominant cell type in CSF	Glucose (mg/100 ml)	Protein (mg/100 ml)
Tuberculosis	20–1,000	Mononuclear	20–80	50–1,000
Fungal (usually) crypto-coccus)	25–500	Mononuclear	20–40	25–500

Parkinsonism (Paralysis Agitans)

I. **Definition.** A progressive neurologic disease affecting primarily the extrapyramidal tracts and characterized by tremor, bradykinesia, rigidity, and festinating gait.

II. **Pathophysiology. Etiologies** include idiopathic as well as postencephalitic and drug-related (phenothiazine, reserpine, manganese, and cobalt poisoning) causes. The **disease mechanism** involves decreased levels of the neurotransmitter dopamine in the basal ganglia (thus the dopamine precursor L-dopa is an effective antiparkinsonian agent) due to degeneration of neuronal tracts in the substantia nigra.

III. **Clinical manifestations.** Parkinsonism usually begins insidiously with a coarse "pill-rolling" resting tremor or "cogwheel rigidity." Gradually other Sx develop: characteristic mask-like facies, festinating gait, bradykinesia. Sx usually respond to antiparkinsonian treatment, but return if the drug is withheld. Long-term control is very difficult to obtain.

IV. **Differential diagnosis.** Dx is made on basis of clinical picture and response to therapy. Tremor of parkinsonism must be distinguished from those of other syndromes, especially senile or essential tremor (familial, faster [9-11/sec], no associated rigidity) and hysterical tremor (increases during stress, decreases during distraction). Always check for phenothiazine usage.

Appendixes

In constrast to the cardiovascular exam, the neurologic exam often receives less emphasis than it deserves. One reason for this is that for the great majority of patients an abbreviated form of the complete neurologic exam is sufficient. In this appendix we provide an outline of a relatively thorough neurologic evaluation annotated with selected clinical points. We emphasize that the complete exam need be done only when there is a suspicion of neurologic disease. For the rest of your patients, the shorter version outlined in Chap. 2 will suffice. The clinical points provided in this appendix may be used as bedside reference material for any questions that arise during your general screening neurologic exam.

I. **Outline of a complete neurologic exam**

   A. **Mental status**

      1. General appearance and behavior

      2. Alertness

      3. Orientation

      4. Memory: recent, remote, recall

      5. Speech

      6. Constructions

      7. Psychiatric appraisal: thought content, insight and judgment, proverbs, affect

      8. Somatic functions: bowel, bladder, sexual

   B. **Cranial nerves**

      1. Olfactory

      2. Optic: fundi, visual activity, visual fields

      3, 4, 6. EOMs

      5. Facial sensation and muscles of mastication

      7. Facial musculature

      8. Auditory-vestibular

      9, 10. Oropharyngeal movements and gag reflex

      11. SCM-trapezius function

      12. Tongue

   C. **Motor system**

      1. Tone, bulk, and power

      2. Tremor, asterixis, and myoclonus

      3. Cerebellar exam

      4. Gait and station

D. Sensory system

1. Pinprick
2. Temperature
3. Position
4. Vibration
5. Light touch
6. "Cortical" discrimination

E. Reflexes

1. Deep tendon reflexes
2. Superficial reflexes
3. Babinski and other pathologic reflexes
4. Developmental reflexes in the infant and child

*F. Neuroskeletal

1. Neck mobility
2. Spine (determine if straight and nontender to percussion)
3. Head circumference in children

*G. Neurovascular

1. Carotid and cranial pulses
2. Ocular and carotid bruits

II. The neurologic exam: selected historical and clinical points

A. Mental status exam. The mental status exam begins any neurologic work-up since interpretation of the rest of the exam depends on it. Remember that many patients you examine will be alert, oriented persons without mental status changes or need for anything more than a quick check to see that they are oriented and attentive. Fig. A-1 portrays the Circle of Willis, illustrating those cerebral arteries commonly affected by stroke. See Chap. 19, Cerebrovascular Disorders, **IV.**

Clinical and historical points

1. General appearance-behavior — Describe patient's dress, grooming, general level of motor activity and responsiveness, facial expressions (or lack of same), grimaces, tics, frequent movements, chain-smoking, cooperation.

2. Alertness — Decide whether patient is alert, lethargic, stuporous, or comatose. This is worth stating in **every work-up.**

3. Orientation-attention — Check orientation to:
   a. **Person** (names of family member or examiner)
   b. **Place** (e.g., hospital)
   c. **Time** (day, month, year)

   Disorientation suggests dementia or organic brain syndromes.

4. Memory — **Recall:** give patient 3 items to remember, explain you will ask for them in 5 minutes, and then do so.

*Findings to be considered in select patients.

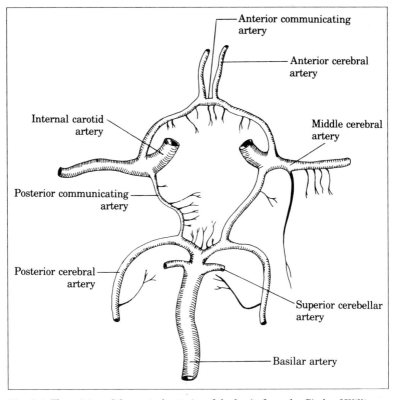

Fig. A-1. The origins of the central arteries of the brain from the Circle of Willis.

Historical points
Recent: inquire about occurrences of last 24 hours; ask for home address and telephone number.
Remote: ask for birthdate, educational and social background, occupation, names of important figures (e.g., high school principal), date of marriage.

5. Speech

Listen for any unusual characteristics or changes in flow; notice the rate.

Check reading and writing if you are seeing an aphasic or confused patient.

Note the presence of unusual words or neologisms.

6. Constructions

Have patient draw a house or cube (not a routine portion of the exam but useful if impairment of cortical function or nondominant hemisphere disease is suspected).

7. Psychiatric appraisal

Note: A formal psychiatric mental status exam is somewhat different and more complete than what is outlined here; it is done in cases of suspected psychiatric illness.

a. Thought content

Note any evidence of hallucinations, delusions, or illusions; note also loose or tangential associations.

b. Insight, judgment

Ask what patient would do if he or she found a stamped, addressed envelope on the street or if a fire broke out in a crowded theatre.

c. Proverbs

Literal interpretation is classically present in psychotic patients (e.g., schizophrenics).

Ask patient to explain the meaning of "A stitch in time saves nine," "Don't count your chickens before they're hatched," "A rolling stone gathers no moss," etc.

d. Affect

Possible alterations include flat or blunted, labile, anxious, angry, depressed, sad, or euphoric.

Ask how the patient is feeling to gain some insight into this issue (mood and affect are closely related).

8. Somatic functions

Ask about bladder and bowel function (continence is a difficult and important issue in neurologic patients).

Ask about sexual function and history of impotence or sexual difficulties.

B. Cranial nerves
   1. Olfactory nerve

Not routinely tested in general exam.

Remember that we are testing **functions,** not isolated components of the neurologic pathway. Malfunction may be at brainstem level, but is may also be due to cerebral, peripheral nerve, or end-organ dysfunction.

Use **nonirritating scents** (e.g., tobacco, wintergreen) and occlude other nostril.

Significant if unilateral loss is present.

Bilateral loss is usually due to trauma or rhinitis.

Historical points
Patients are often unaware of loss, especially unilateral loss.

May complain of no taste.

Olfactory hallucinations suggest temporal lobe disease.

Ask for H/O deviated septum, rhinitis, fracture, other infections.

2. Optic nerve
  a. Visual acuity

Reflects macular vision; test with a pocket Snellen chart or newspaper; test each eye separately; test with patient wearing glasses.

Historical points
Blurred or dim vision.

Night blindness.

  b. Visual fields

Test each eye separately by confrontation as a screening test (order formal perimetry if questionable).

Historical points
Difficulty reading, bumping into things on one side, or blind spots

Patients are often unaware of smaller field cuts.

  c. Pupillary size (afferent limb)

Historical points
See **6.b.**

3. Occulomotor nerve
4. Trochlear nerve
5. Trigeminal nerve
  a. Motor

Palpate masseters on forced closure of jaw.

Check for jaw deviation on forced opening.

Historical points
Jaw fatigue, chewing difficulties.

  b. Corneal response
  c. Sensory

Touch cornea, not sclera, when testing.
Test pin, temperature, and touch on all three divisions of trigeminal.

Historical points
Altered sensation when washing, shaving, drinking, etc.

6. Abducens nerve
  a. Extraocular movements (nerves III, IV, and VI)

Test EOMs on command and patient's ability to follow your finger.

Check for nystagmus as the patient's eyes track and rest.

Historical points
Double vision (diplopia) or blurring.

  b. Pupillary size and reactions

Test direct and consensual response to light.

Lesions may be afferent or efferent.

If you note anisocoria, ask about eyedrop use or long-standing presence.

Historical points
New onset blurring, light sensitivity.

  c. Lid elevation

Examine and compare the widths of the palpebral fissures.

If a fissure is narrowed, consider an ipsilateral Horner's syndrome or a contralateral nerve VII problem.

Ptosis can be oculomotor or sympathetic in origin (the latter tends to be a partial ptosis, with approximately a one-third closure).

Historical points
Check against old snapshots if questionable.

Ask the family if a ptosis is new or old.

7. Facial nerve
   a. Motor

Test facial expressions (smile, grimace), strength of eye closure, width of palpebral fissures, symmetry of nasolabial folds, and forehead wrinkling.

In upper motor neuron (UMN) lesions of nerve VII, the forehead is mostly spared.

UMN (central) lesions are contralateral to any weakness; lower motor neuron (LMN) (peripheral) lesions are ipsilateral to any weakness.

Historical points
Symptomatic complaints of "pulling" of face to opposite side; drooling; "numbness"; thick speech.

   b. Taste (anterior two-thirds of tongue)

Not routinely tested unless peripheral facial lesion or another CN abnormality exists.

Deficits (usually with facial weakness) indicate nerve VII lesion proximal to the chorda tympani.

Test with salt, sugar on a cotton tip applicator.

Historical points
Patients are usually not aware of change.

8. Auditory nerve
   a. Auditory

Use 256- or 512-cps tuning fork for testing low frequency, ticking watch for testing high frequency, whispered voice for testing middle frequency.

Test air vs. bone conduction:
(1) Rinne's test. Bone louder than air indicates a conduction loss.
(2) Weber's test (lateralization of bone conduction from forehead). Sound lateralizes to the side of decreased air conduction (this test is not specific and is often equivocal).

   b. Vestibular

Test gait, check for nystagmus.

Historical points
Dizziness, staggering, vertigo.

9, 10. Glossopharyngeal and vagus nerves

Test swallowing (with water) and phonation ("me," "la," and "ga" for lips, anterior palate, and posterior palate, respectively). Use a tongue depressor to check for a gag reflex.

Nasal speech or lax palate suggest a LMN lesion.

Palate and uvula may be chronically asymmetric, especially if the patient has had a tonsillectomy.

Clear fluids are hardest to handle in most neuromuscular disorders.

Taste on the posterior one-third of the tongue is not routinely tested.

Historical points
Change in voice, clarity of speech, or excessive coughing with food or drink.

11. Spinal accessory nerve

Test shrug (trapezius), turning of head (contralateral sternocleidomastoid [SCM]), and flexion of head (both SCMs).

Historical points
"Wry" neck, head tilt.

12. Hypoglossal nerve

Test for symmetry in protrusion of tongue, strength in pushing tongue out against cheeks, and lingual muscle mass; look for tongue fasciculations.

Minor deviations are often within normal limits.

Some "restlessness" or minor undulations of the resting tongue are normal.

Look for significant fasciculations or weakness possibly associated with atrophy.

Patients are usually unaware of a nerve XII lesion. Occasional difficulty in speech or manipulation of food in mouth occurs.

C. Motor system
1. Muscle strength

Consider degree of cooperation, muscle bulk and condition, and overall condition.

Use the following scale for each muscle group tested and record the patient's best performance.

$0 = 0\%$ = no evidence of contractility

$1 = 10\%$ = trace contractility with no joint motion

$2 = 25\%$ = complete motion with gravity eliminated

$3 = 50\%$ = barely complete motion against gravity

4 = 75% = complete motion against gravity and some resistance

5 = 100% = complete motion against gravity and full resistance

Historical points
Mild weakness may be called "heaviness or numbness."

Weakness may be functionally reported (clumsiness, tripping, dropping things).

Ask about specific functional problems (combing hair, climbing steps, clumsiness, trouble writing) and when during the day trouble is worst.

2. Muscle tone

Resistance to passive motion is tested first.

Decreased tone is hard to detect; an impression of floppiness or laxity may emerge.

Patient must be relaxed to examine tone.

Common causes of increased tone include:
a. Difficulty relaxing (anxiety, gegenhalten).
b. Spasticity (extremity opens suddenly like a clasp knife).
c. Extrapyramidal (including "cogwheeling").

Parkinsonian characteristics:
Expressionless facies, resting tremor ("pill rolling"), shuffling gait, cogwheel rigidity, and bradykinesia.

Historical points
Patients are generally unaware of mild increases of tone; they may complain of aching, especially at night.

More severe rigidity may be noted as tightness, aching, cramping, stiffening, or curling up.

3. Muscle bulk

Allow for handedness, occupational, or exercise-induced differences.

Compare one side of the body to the other: palpate muscles at rest and when contracting; measure for differences.

Look for fasciculations.

Atrophy is c/w disuse and nutritional, neurogenic, or late-stage myopathic etiologies.

Check for associated signs of inflammation or tenderness.

Historical points
Patients may note wasting, but often will not be good witnesses to the time course.

D. Sensory system
1. Pinprick

Use (with prudence) head of pin vs. point of pin for "dull" vs. "sharp."

Distal extremity testing is usually adequate for screening in the absence of symptoms.

If decreased sensation is noted, test more proximally and locate point at which impairment begins.

Compare proximal and distal, right and left pinpricks.

Historical points
Impairment is frequently unnoticed by patient. Ask for unnoticed burns, cuts, or poorly healing ulcers.

The patient may complain of burning, searing, hot, or cold sensations in areas (**paresthesias**).

2. Temperature

Compare temperature of a tuning fork ("cold") to that of the rubber of a reflex hammer ("warm").

Generally coincides with pinprick sensation (see Fig. A-2), but one may be altered out of proportion to the other.

Altered temperature is sometimes easier to detect than pinprick.

Historical points
Altered sense of shaving, bathing, dishwater, or hot or cold drinks may be reported.

Impairments are often unnoticed by patients.

3. Position

Move toe up or down, asking the patient to describe direction in which you have moved it; grasp the sides of the toe tested to avoid giving pressure cues.

Romberg's test applies to this system (does loss of visual cues lead to instability?): ask patient to stand and close eyes; and then observe stability.

Joint position sense tests only part of proprioception and may be normal in a patient with, for example, a positive Romberg.

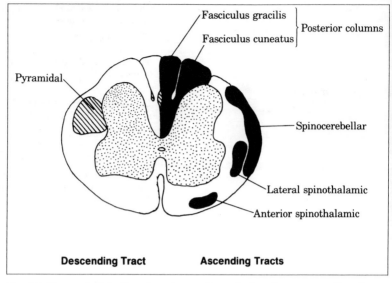

Fig. A-2. The most clinically relevant ascending spinal cord tracts, as well as the crucial descending tract, the pyramidal tract, are shown. Recall that each ascending tract is predominantly concerned with a sensory modality: the posterior columns with position and vibration sense as well as stereognosis, the lateral spinothalamic tract with pain and temperature, the anterior spinothalamic tract with tactile sense, and the spinocerebellar tracts with proprioception and stereognosis. The pyramidal tract is the major descending motor system.

Historical points
Trouble walking, perhaps greatest at night or on rough ground.

Foot-slapping, general clumsiness, or impaired facility not obviously related to weakness are all possible symptoms of decreased position sense.

4. Vibration
Use 128- or 256-cps tuning fork.

Joint position sense (see **3**) involves discriminative functions and, if vibratory sense is much better, abnormal position sense may indicate parietal dysfunction.

Be sure the patient is distinguishing vibration as opposed to pressure from the fork (check this with a "sham" vibration caused by pressing the extremity with the end of the nonvibrating fork).

Historical points
No specific symptoms.

Posterior column (see Fig. A-2) symptoms in general may include feelings of

5. Light touch

tightness, envelopment, or constriction. Also "pins and needles" sensation or numbness may be reported.

Use cotton wisp, e.g., from the end of a cotton tip applicator.

A cooperative patient can often help locate involved areas by running a cotton wisp or hand lightly along the trunk or extremity.

Historical points
May have posterior column symptoms (see above).

May note impaired feeling in course of normal self-touch.

6. "Cortical" discrimination

Testing examples include:
a. Graphesthesia, the perception of letter or number writing on digit, palm, sole, etc.
b. Somatesthesia, the manual recognition of comb or coin with eyes closed.
c. Two-point discrimination, which can be used if paralysis or paresis are present, as can graphesthesia, since these tests do not require motor participation.

Note: Impaired touch sensation renders these tests virtually useless.

E. Reflexes
1. Deep tendon reflexes
   a. Biceps (C5,6)
   b. Triceps (C6,7,8)
   c. Brachioradialis (C5,6)
   d. Knee jerk (patellar) (L2,3,4)
   e. Ankle jerk (Achilles) (S1,2)

Limbs should be relaxed and well supported; distraction and/or the reinforcement technique may help. Do not be fooled by the passive movement of the tendon by the hammer.

Deep tendon reflexes (DTRs) are usually graded on a scale of 1–4, with 1+ = difficult to elicit but present (with or without augmentation technique); 2+ = average; 3+ = hyperactive but not necessarily pathologic; 4+ = very hyperactive with associated clonus (usually pathological). Also note the time necessary for the relaxation phase (increased, for example, in hypothyroidism).

2. Superficial reflexes
   a. Corneal

See Cranial Nerve V discussion above.

   b. Abdominals
      (1) Upper (T7,8,9)
      (2) Lower (T11,12)

Stroke out or across the four periumbilical quadrants.

   c. Cremasteric (T12,L1)

In general decreased contralateral to acute pyramidal lesions, temporarily.

Abdominal reflexes are useful in suspected spinal cord lesions and can help to establish level of involvement.
Abdominal reflexes may be hard to

3. Pathologic reflexes
   a. Plantar responses

elicit, and may be absent if a paramedian incision or scars are present.

Abdominal and cremasteric reflexes tend to fatigue quickly on repeated elicitation. Cremasterics are only rarely helpful.

(Extension or flexion of great toe occurs on lateral plantar stimulation.)

Stroke plantar surface **laterally** to minimize withdrawal and to avoid a plantar "grasp."

The **Babinski sign** is the pathologic **extensor plantar** response.

Extensor response with triple flexion of the leg may be hard at times to differentiate from voluntary withdrawal. Voluntary withdrawal is rarely purely flexor; often a more complex "shaking-off" is involved.

Note: Grasping, sucking, and rooting—the "primitive" or "release" reflexes listed below—generally signify frontal lobe dysfunction. They may be initiated by visual as well as tactile stimuli.

   b. Grasp (palm or sole)

Gently stroke your hand along the patient's palm.

Stroke along the palm toward the patient's fingertips, which may elicit tugging by the patient's flexed fingers.

   c. Suck, root

Touch stimulation of the lips produces pursing (suck); touching the corners of the patient's mouth and cheek produces head turning and lip groping toward the stimulus.

4. Bilateral cortico-bulbar reflexes

Pouting of lips occurs if examiner's finger is drawn across the patient's lips or if the perioral area is lightly tapped.

   a. Jaw jerk

Light downward tap on a finger placed on the patient's chin leads to a reflexive jerk of the jaw.

5. Extrapyramidal reflex, glabellar

Repetitive finger taps in the region between the patient's eyebrows causes reflex in patients with Parkinson's disease (i.e., repetitive eye blinking that does not extinguish).

Historical points

A positive (abnormal) test is the relative failure to inhibit the blink in response to this repetitive stimulus.

6. *Other* reflexes
   a. Startle myoclonus

Sudden unexpected clap, turning on of light, tap on body creates a "startle" response. (A local or mass **myoclonic reaction** is a response to sudden tactile, visual, or auditory stimuli; it generally indicates neuronal "hyperirritability," as in withdrawal syndromes and certain neuronal disease.)

b. Oculocephalic

"Doll's eyes" response to a quick, passive turn of the patient's head. (The reflex is mediated by vestibular and neck proprioceptive receptors; it is minimally present in alert patients but is present in stuporous or comatose patients with **intact brainstem tegmental connections.**)

c. Ciliospinal

Pinch lateral neck of comatose patient and observe the pupil. (Pupillary dilatation in response to pinch on neck is sympathetically mediated; it may work in patients with Horner's disease.)

d. Anal wink

A light scratch is made on perianal skin; this is a segmental reflex to demonstrate intactness of lower motor neuron.

Appendix B

Common Serum Chemistries

Test	Current units	Factor[a]	SI units
Albumin	3.5–4.8 gm/100 ml	.154	0.54–0.74 mmol/l
Ammonia (plasma)	18–48 μg/100 ml	.587	10.6–28.2 μmol/l
Bilirubin			
Total	.25–1.5 mg/100 ml[b]	17.1	4.3–25.6 μmol/l
Direct	0–.2 mg/100 ml		0–3.4 μmol/l
Blood gases (arterial, whole blood)			
pH	7.35–7.45	1	7.35–7.45
PO_2	80–105 mm Hg	.133	10.6–14.0 kPa
PCO_2	35–45 mm Hg	.133	4.7–6.0 kPa
Calcium			
Total	9.0–10.3 mg/100 ml	.25	2.25–2.57 mmol/l
Free[c]	4.5–5.0 mg/100 ml	.25	1.12–1.25 mmol/l
Carbon dioxide content	24–32 mEq/L	1	24–32 mmol/l
Beta-carotene	70–250 μg/100 ml	.0186	1.3–4.6 μmol/l
Ceruloplasmin	15–60 mg/100 ml	.067	1.0–4.0 μmol/l
Chloride	95–105 mEq/L	1	95–105 mmol/l
Copper	70–155 μg/100 ml[b]	.157	11.0–24.3 μmol/l
Complement (total)[d]	150–250 CH50	1	150–250 arb. units
C3	690–1,470 mg/L	.001	0.7–1.5 g/l
C4	105–305 mg/L	.001	0.10–0.30 g/l
Creatinine			
Male	.8–1.3 mg/100 ml	88.4	71–115 μmol/l
Female	.6–1.1 mg/100 ml		53–97 μmol/l
Fibrinogen[e]	1.5–3.6 gm/L	1	1.5–3.6 g/l
Folate			
Serum[f]	>3 ng/ml	2.27	>6.81 nmol/l
Red cell	117–541 ng/ml		226–1,228 nmol/l

[a]A complete list of multiplication factors for converting conventional units to SI units can be found in *N. Engl. J. Med.* 292:795, 1975.
[b]Variation with age and sex occurs. This range includes both sexes and persons >13 years old.
[c]Performed by an ion-selective electrode technique.
[d]Reported as CH50: the reciprocal of the dilution of sera required to lyse 50% of sheep erythrocytes.
[e]Determined by the Clauss method.
[f]Competitive protein binding assay using beta-lactoglobulin.
[g]The units for quantitating immunoglobulins are not agreed on. They are arbitrarily expressed here as grams per liter as determined by radial immunodiffusion. The normal ranges for blacks include substantially higher values.
[h]Because of the variable composition of serum triglycerides, their concentration is expressed here as grams rather than moles per liter. A mean molecular weight of 875 gm has also been used. Varies with age.
[i]In the International System, serum protein concentrations determined by electrophoresis are expressed as g/l.
Source: From Department of Medicine, Washington University School of Medicine, *Manual of Medical Therapeutics* (23rd ed.), edited by J. F. Freitag and L. W. Miller. Boston: Little, Brown, 1980.

Test	Current units	Factor[a]	SI units
Glucose, fasting (plasma)	65–110 mg/100 ml	.055	3.57–6.05 mmol/l
Haptoglobin	100–300 mg/100 ml	.01	1.10–3.00 g/l
Immunoglobulin[g]			
IgA	39–358 mg/100 ml	.01	0.39–3.58 g/l
IgM	33–229 mg/100 ml	.01	0.33–2.29g/l
IgG	679–1,537 mg/100 ml	.01	6.79–15.37 g/l
Iron			
Male	80–160 μg/100 ml	.179	14.3–28.6 μmol/l
Female	60–135 μg/100 ml		10.7–24.2 μmol/l
Binding capacity	250–350 μg/100 ml		44.7–62.6 μmol/l
Lactate (plasma)	.3–1.3 mmol/L	1	0.3–1.3 mmol/l
Lipids			
Cholesterol[b]	120–330 mg/100 ml	.0259	3.1–8.5 mmol/l
Triglyceride[b,h]	10–190 mg/100 ml	.01	0.1–1.9 g/l
Magnesium	1.5–2.4 mEq/L	.5	0.7–1.2 mmol/l
Osmolality	270–290 mOsm/kg	1	270–290 mOsm/kg
Phosphorus, inorganic[b]	2.5–6.0 mg/100 ml	.323	0.8–1.9 mmol/l
Potassium (plasma)	3.5–4.5 mEq/L	1	3.5–4.5 mmol/l
Protein electrophoresis[i]			
Albumin	3.5–4.8 gm/100 ml	10	35–48 g/l
Alpha-1-globulin	0.1–0.5 gm/100 ml	10	1–5 g/l
Alpha-2-globulin	0.3–1.2 gm/100 ml	10	3–12 g/l
Beta-globulin	0.7–1.7 gm/100 ml	10	7–17 g/l
Gamma-globulin	0.7–1.7 gm/100 ml	10	7–17 g/l
Protein total	6.5–8.5 gm/100 ml	10	65–85 g/l
Pyruvate (whole blood)	30–70 μmol/L	1	30–70 μmol/l
Sodium	135–145 mEq/L	1	135–145 mmol/l
Urea nitrogen[b]	12–30 mg/100 ml	.357	4.3–10.7 mmol/l
Uric acid[b]	3.5–8.0 mg/100 ml	.059	0.21–0.47 mmol/l
Vitamin A	30–65 μg/100 ml	.035	1.05–2.27 μmol/l
Vitamin B_{12}	250–1,000 pg/ml	.739	185–739 pmol/l

[a]A complete list of multiplication factors for converting conventional units to SI units can be found in *N. Engl. J. Med.* 292:795, 1975.
[b]Variation with age and sex occurs. This range includes both sexes and persons >13 years old.
[c]Performed by an ion-selective electrode technique.
[d]Reported as CH50: the reciprocal of the dilution of sera required to lyse 50% of sheep erythrocytes.
[e]Determined by the Clauss method.
[f]Competitive protein binding assay using beta-lactoglobulin.
[g]The units for quantitating immunoglobulins are not agreed on. They are arbitrarily expressed here as grams per liter as determined by radial immunodiffusion. The normal ranges for blacks include substantially higher values.
[h]Because of the variable composition of serum triglycerides, their concentration is expressed here as grams rather than moles per liter. A mean molecular weight of 875 gm has also been used. Varies with age.
[i]In the International System, serum protein concentrations determined by electrophoresis are expressed as g/l.
Source: From Department of Medicine, Washington University School of Medicine, *Manual of Medical Therapeutics* (23rd ed.), edited by J. F. Freitag and L. W. Miller. Boston: Little, Brown, 1980.

Most students do not buy clinical texts wisely. There is a tendency either to buy no books at all or to buy every text that looks as though it might someday be useful. The following list represents what we consider to be a core clinical library of books that every student should either own or borrow. More information on the authors and publishers of these books can be found in the References that follow.

I. **Medical dictionary.** Good medical dictionaries actually resemble one-volume medical encyclopedias, with good illustrations and cross-references. A good exercise is to look up the entries under the subject "signs" and to skim through the many diagnostic points contained in this section.

   We recommend *Dorland's Illustrated Medical Dictionary*. It is prefaced by an especially good section on medical etymology.

II. **Major medical textbooks.** Although these are expensive, we recommend that the student buy two:

   A. **Harvey's** is probably the best introductory text. It is well organized, eminently readable, and easy to digest. Its many tables and diagrams are especially good and are worth copying for your personal "black book."

   B. **Harrison's** still sets the standard for comprehensive medical textbooks. Most medical students learn to appreciate it more and more as they gain clinical experience.

III. **Brief summaries and overviews.** These books are good introductions and reviews. They are useful to keep in your locker for those times when you need a 5-minute consult or a starting point for your case reading:

   A. *Current Medical Diagnosis and Treatment* is a telegraphic paperback emphasizing clinical manifestations and diagnosis.

   B. *Medicine* is a highly readable, pathophysiologically oriented summary of diagnosis and treatment of the most common diseases. Compiled by five house officers at the Massachusetts General Hospital, this is a good book to read in your first couple of months on the wards.

IV. **Books to carry on the wards**

   A. *Manual of Medical Therapeutics.* Just as the name implies, this paperback is an up-to-date summary of medical treatments. If you carry only one book, this should be it. Like all the spiral manuals, it is pitched at exactly the right level for the student or intern.

   B. *Problem-Oriented Medical Diagnosis.* This book is a handy guide to the work-ups of the most common medical problems. The lists of differential diagnoses and diagnostic algorithms can be real time-savers.

   C. *Practical Guide to the Care of the Surgical Patient.* This small handbook of useful information is the original "peripheral brain." The telegraphic section on common drugs is especially useful.

   D. *Manual of Clinical Problems in Internal Medicine.* Read the pertinent sections in this book just before you present your case on rounds. They will give you an idea of current issues and controversies in diagnosis and management.

V. Physical diagnosis

    A. Bates is probably the best physical diagnosis text for the total novice. Its diagrams and brevity make it easy to absorb. However, many students choose to borrow rather than purchase it because its useful lifetime is only a few months.

    B. DeGowin and DeGowin is complete and authoritative, although many parts may be too detailed for the second-year student.

VI. Clinical laboratory

    A. *Serum Chemistry and Hematology: Wallach's Interpretation of Diagnostic Tests* contains reasonably complete lists of most serum chemistry and hematology results. This book is often too complete to be really useful, but you will find it an aid in constructing your differential diagnosis list.

    B. ECG interpretation. We recommend three books:

        1. Dubin is a very simple and straightforward approach to ECG interpretation. Try to borrow rather than buy it, because you will absorb it in a few evenings.

        2. Mudge has the best collection of abnormal ECGs of any introductory text. The unknowns are particularly useful.

        3. Marriott is the definitive introductory ECG book. Good for the advanced student.

    C. Radiology. Squires is the classic introductory text of diagnostic radiology. Every student should read it.

VII. Other texts

    A. *Atlas of Bedside Procedures* is the best of the (illustrated) "how-to" books.

    B. *Renal and Electrolyte Disorders* is a concise but comprehensive treatment of a traditionally difficult area. The sections on acid-base disorders are particularly good.

    C. *Neurology for the House Officer* is a small paperback that presents a brief summary of most common neurologic problems.

    D. *Cope's Early Diagnosis of the Acute Abdomen* is the classic text on clinical evaluation of tender bellies.

References

Note: For our recommendations concerning the most useful book(s) in various areas, see Appendix C.

1. Adams, F. *Physical Diagnosis* (14th ed). Baltimore: Williams & Wilkins, 1958.
2. Alpert, J., and Rippe, J. *Manual of Cardiovascular Diagnosis and Therapy*. Boston: Little, Brown, 1980.
3. Bates, B. *A Guide to Physical Examination* (2nd ed). Philadelphia: Lippincott, 1979.
4. Beeson, P., and McDermott, W. (Eds.) *Cecil-Loeb Textbook of Medicine* (16th ed). Philadelphia: Saunders, 1982.
5. Campbell, J., and Frisse, M. (Eds.). *Manual of Medical Therapeutics* (24th ed). Boston: Little, Brown, 1983.
6. DeGowin E, and DeGowin, R. *Bedside Diagnostic Examination* (3rd ed). New York: Macmillan, 1976.
7. Delp, M., and Manning, R. (Eds.) *Major's Physical Diagnosis: An Introduction to the Clinical Process* (9th ed.). Philadelphia: Saunders, 1981.
8. Dubin, D. *Rapid Interpretation of EKG's: a Programmed Course*. Tampa, Fla.: Cover Publishing, 1974.
9. Federman, D., and Rubenstein, E. (Eds.). *Scientific American Medicine*. New York: Scientific American, 1978.
10. Fishman, M., Hoffman, A., Klausner, R., Rockson, S., and Thaler, M. *Medicine*. Philadelphia: Lippincott, 1981.
11. Folstein, M., et al. *J. Psychiatr. Res.* 12:189–198, 1975.
12. Friedman, H. (Ed.). *Problem-Oriented Medical Diagnosis* (2nd ed). Boston: Little, Brown, 1979.
13. Goldberg, M., et al. *J.A.M.A.* 223(3):269–275, 1973.
14. Harrell, R., and Firestein, G. *The Effective Scutboy*. New York: Arco Publishing, 1981.
15. Harvey, A., et al. (Eds.). *The Principles and Practice of Medicine* (20th ed). New York; McGraw-Hill, 1980.
16. Hochstein, E., and Rubin, A. *Physical Diagnosis*. New York: McGraw-Hill, 1964.
17. Isselbacher, K., et al. (Eds.). *Harrison's Principles of Internal Medicine* (9th ed). New York; McGraw-Hill, 1980.
18. Judge, R., and Zuidema, G. *Methods of Clinical Examination: A Physiologic Approach*. Boston: Little, Brown, 1974.
19. Kapff, C., and Jandl, J. *Blood: Atlas and Sourcebook of Hematology*. Boston: Little, Brown, 1981.
20. Krupp, M., et al. (Eds.). *Physician's Handbook* (19th ed). Los Altos, Calif.: Lange, 1979.
21. Krupp, M., and Chatton, M. (Eds.). *Current Medical Diagnosis and Treatment*. Los Altos, Calif.: Lange, 1981.
22. Marriott, H. *Practical Electrocardiography* (6th ed). Baltimore: Williams & Wilkins, 1977.
23. McEntyre, R. *Practical Guide to the Care of the Surgical Patient*. St. Louis: Mosby, 1980.
24. Morgan, W., and Engel, G. *The Clinical Approach to the Patient*. Philadelphia: Saunders, 1969.
25. Mudge, G. *Manual of Electrocardiography*. Boston: Little, Brown, 1981.
26. Portlock, R., and Goffret, M. *Manual of Clinical Problems in Oncology*. Boston: Little, Brown, 1980.
27. Reich, P. *Hematology*. Boston: Little, Brown, 1978.

28. Schrier, R. *Renal and Electrolyte Disorders.* Boston: Little, Brown, 1980.
29. Silen, W. (Ed.). *Cope's Early Diagnosis of the Acute Abdomen* (15th ed). New York: Oxford University Press, 1979.
30. Snell, R. *Clinical Anatomy for Medical Students* (2nd ed). Boston: Little, Brown, 1981.
31. Spivak, J., and Barnes, H. *Manual of Clinical Problems in Internal Medicine* (2nd ed). Boston: Little, Brown, 1978.
32. Squires, L. *Fundamentals of Radiology* (rev. ed.). Cambridge, Mass.: Harvard University Press, 1975.
33. Stein, J. H. *Internal Medicine.* Boston: Little, Brown, 1983.
34. Troupin, R. *Diagnostic Radiology in Clinical Medicine* (2nd ed). Chicago: Year Book, 1978.
35. Walker, H., et al. (Eds.). *Clinical Methods: The History, Physical and Laboratory Examinations.* Boston: Butterworth, 1976.
36. Wallach, J. *Interpretation of Diagnostic Tests: A Handbook of Laboratory Medicine* (3rd ed). Boston: Little, Brown, 1978.
37. Vandersalm, T., Cutler, B., and Wheeler, H. *Atlas of Bedside Procedures.* Boston: Little, Brown, 1979.

References, Unpublished

1. Coggins, C. Urinalysis. Harvard Medical School, Renal Pathophysiology Handouts.
2. Funkenstein, H., and Glick, T. Approach to the Neurologic Patient. Harvard Medical School, Introduction to Clinical Medicine Handout.
3. Harvard Medical School, Pathophysiology Handouts.

Index

Index